Health Dynamics

A Unique Principle of Self-Healing

Christiane Vée

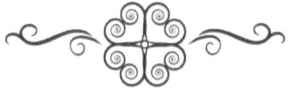

First published by Busybird Publishing 2017
Copyright © 2017 Christiane Vée

ISBN
Print: 978-1-925692-92-1
Ebook: 978-1-925692-44-0

Christiane Vée has asserted her right under the Copyright, Designs and Patents Act 1988 to be identified as the author of this work. The information in this book is based on the author's experiences and opinions. The publisher specifically disclaims responsibility for any adverse consequences, which may result from use of the information contained herein. Permission to use information has been sought by the author. Any breaches will be rectified in further editions of the book.

All rights reserved. No part of this publication may be reproduced, stored in or introduced into a retrieval system, or transmitted in any form, or by any means (electronic, mechanical, photocopying, recording or otherwise) without the prior written permission of the author. Any person who does any unauthorised act in relation to this publication may be liable to criminal prosecution and civil claims for damages. Enquiries should be made through the publisher.

Cover image: Elena Vaseo, AEV Photography
Cover design: Kev Howlett, Busybird
Ilustrations: Alyca Amery
Layout and typesetting: Busybird Publishing:

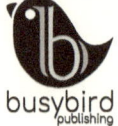

Busybird Publishing
2/118 Para Road
Montmorency, Victoria
Australia 3094
www.busybird.com.au

DISCLAIMER: This book is intended to supplement, not replace, the advice of a trained healthcare practitioner. If you know or suspect that you have a health problem, please consult a healthcare practitioner. The publisher specifically disclaims responsibility for any adverse consequences, which may result from the use of the information contained within this book.

Testimonials

'Christiane Vée has been a strong stalwart leader who has refused to give in to her character and has lead others in declaring herself as a leader. She is a genuine, caring person who has always put others first. She has taken on jobs fearlessly well outside her usual responsibilities. She continues to seek more knowledge and take actions that will give her what she desires despite her doubts. I have no problems in endorsing her as someone who is exceptional and with the highest integrity.'

    Kerry Parry
*   Head Coach, Introduction Leader Program,* **Landmark Education**

'Christiane is always very professional. Her commitment to helping me, listening to me, and mentoring me has been enlightening, full of fun and inspiration, and always with a smile. All the work modules were clear and easy to follow and I knew Christiane would explain anything if needed at any time. She made herself available and was always flexible when my work commitments become so busy. I love the clarity of our time and knew it was confidential and I could be myself and in being open and honest I knew I would get non-judgemental guidance and support.'

    Dianne Hayman
*   Owner/Manager,* **Great Expectations**

'Over the past 6 years Christiane has worked with me as my Life Coach. During that time, my life has transformed! From where I was then to where I am now is a complete blessing! Her intuitive manner helped me tremendously when I was distressed! She knew when to be gentle and when she could be firm. She helped to keep me on track, moving forward – something that gave me clarity and direction. Every aspect of my life has improved and having Christiane in my life is a blessing!'

    Tracey Korman
*   Managing Director,* **Two's Company**

'What has changed since the coaching is making things clear – no bias, a contribution which enabled me to not worry and be anxious too much. Being available when I usually needed someone to listen and to assure me that this is what happens when life is working. Someone to bounce off – a sounding board on what's happening to make better decisions. Being straight with me – to get real – to get results.'

    Gina Campion
    Anyinginyi Health Aboriginal Corporation

'I have known Christiane Vée for more than 10 years and she never ceases to amaze me. She has been my coach, mentor, friend, colleague, and has been the main person I have called on when I have been stuck with an issue. Every time, she has helped me move through it with grace and ease. I wish her every success with her book and hope that it inspires everyone who reads it to be the best they can be.'

    Aldwyn Altuney
    Photojournalist/Director, Xposé Media

'I met Christiane when she was a client of mine many years ago and straight away I could see that Christiane had a big heart and something special to offer the world. She is passionate about helping others reach their potential, not just in health but in life. Christiane, through the example of her own life, shows we all have the potential to transform. We just have to believe it and take the necessary steps.'

    Mireille Ryan
    Social Media Strategist

'In my long pursuit for optimal health, I have consumed countless articles and books on the topic. However, Christiane Vée's *Health Dynamics: A Unique Principle of Self-Healing* stands out as a refreshing and authentic insight into both the mental and physical aspects of health. It is always reassuring when an author embodies such written principles to great success, and Christiane is a perfect example of that. Her adventurous and free-spirited attitude towards life is nothing short of inspiring. It is therefore no surprise that her blueprint for success lives up to her own reputation.'

Sam Saffuri
Intouch Massage Chairs

'I fled my toxic and dangerous life with my ex. Your love and contribution single-handedly scooped me up and transported me to a safe place that I discovered in myself and you guided me to this magical sanctum. Thank you for being a most extraordinary human and friend and coach. Your contribution means so much and instils so much for me. You have restored my faith in myself and men and humanity.'

Kacey Holden

To Christophe, my son, Tyler, my grandson, and Phil, my best friend who is totally dedicated to me – I feel blessed!

To my mother, Arlette, who was highly spiritual and full of wisdom.

To Mireille Ryan who in 2014 suggested I write a book, and Natasa Denman, who believed in my ability to write this book – you really inspire me.

Contents

Introduction	i
Powerful Mind	1
Body Wisdom	11
Our Beliefs	19
Beyond Medication	27
Food Essence	33
Tasty and Wholesome	41
Nurture Yourself	53
Your Quest	61
Time Indulgence	67
Total Transformation	75
Global Shift	83
A conversation with Rudran Brannock	89
Rudran Brannock	103
Afterword	105
References and Other Reading	107
About the Author	109
Sexy Healthy Love It Packages	111
Blockage Relief Session	113

Introduction

Who would have thought that I'd write a book? Not me. For years I told myself that one day I would write a book, but the more I thought about it, the more unattainable it seemed. So, this is a dream come true and a complete miracle for me. Although I had it on my vision board all last year, I did not know how it was going to happen. It not only took the right person, Natasa, to have me believe that it was possible, but she also made sure that I followed up with it.

I met Natasa briefly at a business expo in 2016. I was impressed by her 'down to earth' attitude. I got the brochures and she asked for my business card. She said that she was giving a prize away and that she would let me know the result. I thought it would be unlikely that I'd hear from her again. The ticket was to be drawn on Facebook Live, but I was not the winner. Thinking about it now, I realise that not winning the prize was fine because I ended up winning the special connection with Natasa. Nat is unstoppable and she makes you see that 'if you do the work you will get the result'. She helped make my dream a reality.

When I decided I was going to write this book, I did not know what the title would be. I had so much in my head that I wanted to get it all out and share with others. We can sometime write a book in our head but it takes a different shape. It becomes clearer and more specific when we end up putting it on paper. It is even better in a book because you can have more people reading about your story. Then it is not about you, but about how it resonates with the reader. They see themselves in your story because they had a similar experience.

Once I committed to this, it all came back to me that when I was in high school I had wanted to write a book, and have a pen name. We had a teacher who was filling in for our French teacher, and I was so impressed by the way she spoke. She was Chinese and spoke impeccable French, and the lesson that day was about pen names. I started dreaming that one day I would be a writer and that my pen name would be her last name. Behold! These crazy dreams that children have can and do become a reality in the end, but only if they have the courage to make it happen.

Many years down the track I changed my name because I chose not to be identified with my married name any longer. I was divorced and wanted to leave the past behind. I did not want to go back to my maiden name because then I was a shy, helpless, and fearful girl who had no purpose and was quite vague about life in general. I wanted to be the powerful human being who had bravely come out of an abusive situation. I was determined to carve a new life for myself. I wanted to re-write my life and inspire others to do the same.

I was about to sign some very important documents so I went to the Department of Birth, Deaths, and Marriages in the city, and within four hours I had a new name. The amazing thing about it is that I had unconsciously changed it to my pen name by using the first letter of my maiden name and turning it into a word. It was only when writing this book that I realised that I manifested what I created so many years ago while I was in high school. But back then I had no idea of the circumstances that I would have to go through prior to my name change.

Health is a huge interest of mine, mainly because I survived mental, physical, and emotional abuse. I had to dig deep within myself to restore my life so I could become whole and complete

Introduction

again. I kept connecting with people and got to value my role on the planet. I kept learning about life which gradually took me to higher levels of awakening. I know that I still do not have all the answers. As I go along, new messages keeping unfolding, steering me onto the right path.

Further on in this book I talk about religion, highlighting how, as much as religions differ, they all have messages of love and getting closer to God. We were born in the image of God and get tainted along the way. We then strive to get back to who we were originally. It is like a contract that we have to fulfil while we are here. It is about exiting the planet on a high note. All religions, we hope, are working towards the same purpose – 1000 years of peace on Earth. Religion and traditions have a huge influence on who we end up becoming. As children we cannot make choices for ourselves. Some of us are more sensitive than others. No matter how good or bad life is, we always carry a little fragment of what we see, hear, and experience within us. We play the game of life not knowing how it will pan out.

The idea is to crack the code in order to survive. The real answer is to go with the flow. In other words, accept what is, and then create what you really want for yourself. We can only change something when we accept it. If we resist, oppose, or react to it, we have already lost the battle. It is like swimming against the current; you get taken away, unable to save yourself. This has been a huge lesson in my life, and it took me quite some years to work it out. Once I did, life got smoother and easier.

I was born in a country with diverse cultures and religions. I always wondered where I fit in all of it. We had maids working for us, and I felt bad for them; it seemed that there was a stigma attached to it. From a spiritual point of view, I also had a lot of questions. I always went to schools run by nuns and corporal punishment was still practised. I was regularly hit with the side of a ruler on the bony part of my outstretched hand, and I had to stay back after school as punishment. And yet, we were told to 'never forget that you are Roman Catholics', and that we were a superior religion. I kept asking myself, 'What about the other people who had different religions and still had a good heart'? The judgement of black and white made me very uncomfortable. In God's eyes we are all the same, 'made in His image', but I believe that today this way of thinking has completely changed in the world. Besides, we are all connected. I am so happy that in Australia we can celebrate how different we are and how we can contribute to each other because of that. Coming to live in Australia gave me freedom to become who I wanted to be.

Being influenced by both French and British colonisation while growing up in Mauritius, I feel blessed to speak fluently in both languages. The education system on the island was outstanding.

Being able to write this book is a huge blessing for me. All my life I believed that I was not good enough. My therapist and mentor, Annie, was the first person who gave me hugs, and for the first time I felt loved. During the difficult times in my marriage she had me discover my inner strength and power, claiming a more fulfilling and happier life. I discovered the authentic love within myself and went about discovering the same in others.

Today, I feel that I am constantly surrounded by love wherever I go. I feel truly blessed in my life.

Powerful Mind

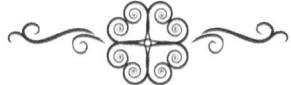

How about training your mind to get the best results in your life?

'The mind is a powerful force. It can enslave us or empower us. It can plunge us into the depths of misery or take us to the heights of ecstasy. Learn to use the power wisely.'
– David Cuschieri

When dealing with a life that does not work, how about assessing what is not working and what needs to be done? This then will open new doors to a multitude of possibilities.

When a thought comes, we don't have to endorse it, but observe the message that it brings. Our thoughts and feelings may come from anywhere from the past. All we have to do it look, listen, and learn. When writing our thoughts or sharing them with others we get better insights about life. So when our thoughts bring up situations that we find difficult to deal with we can make a decision about it, but at the same time be detached from it.

What we think and say creates the world we live in. Being aware of what we think and what we say can manifest itself into a world that is full of peace and happiness.

In contrast:
Some people allow fear to take over their life, and this disempowers them. They wait until life gets better. Life does not get better until we ask for what we want, and do what it takes to get it.

By getting to know who we really are and what we want connects us to the Universe.

We learn to be compassionate towards ourselves and others. We also learn to manage our fears and trust that there is an infinite intelligence we can tap into to provide for us. For some of us, that intelligence is God, our creator. We get to know that we are supported at all times.

What is a thought? What initiates a thought, and where does it come from? Do you think that it is a function of the brain? Of course it is! The brain controls the sensory and motor activities

of the body. This is where all signals are processed to and from the special sense organs related to sight, hearing, taste, smell, and balance. This includes all the main functions of the body, from the beating of the heart, to the blinking of the eye.

A thought is not only a feeling but also an impulse that we experience when we have an idea, a desire to do something like taking a walk on the beach, or eating something. It is an instinct, just like wanting to help someone, or changing something that we do not like. When we have a thought or a feeling, our brain manufactures neuropeptides which are protein-like chemicals. These chemicals act as communicators to other brain cells. As a results these neurotransmitters instantly convey messages to other parts of the body and the whole body responds accordingly. Receptors are located throughout the body ready to receive these communicators. This process allows cells from different parts of the body to speak to each other instantly.

This is the reason why when we experience fear or have feelings of wellbeing and joy it is felt throughout the body. The mind is not isolated to the brain but is in every cell of the body, therefore every cell literally knows our thoughts the moment they happen. When you say to yourself, 'I am so excited' or 'I am sad' your body automatically feels it and creates physiological changes accordingly.

Since these chemical messages can trigger positive or negative responses in our body, we have the power to alter and safeguard our own wellbeing. We can learn to manage the destructive thoughts so our whole being does not get impacted. We can learn to welcome feelings of exuberance or bliss and banish the moody feelings to avoid a space of darkness. The good feelings create chemicals that boost our immune system. A strong immune system helps combat viruses and diseases that may invade our body.

When we have bad thoughts, especially when we are holding on to past experiences, we create toxins in the cells of our body. The type of molecules that our adrenal glands manufacture as a result of anger, resentment, or even anxiety send harmful chemicals throughout the body, depleting the immune system. Such toxic chemicals end up exposing the body and mind to an imbalance and painful conditions.

We create chemicals within the body due to the interpretation of sensory experiences, and these become memories in our body. Most of the time we are totally unaware of this process and how it transforms the body. As these memories manifest themselves in the brain cells, they get encoded before being communicated throughout the body.

Scientists talk about the 'placebo' and the 'nocebo' effects. We can easily evoke a healing response in our body by restructuring the interpretation of what is said or done to us. When referring to the placebo effect the patient is given a non-medicated pill and told that this will improve their condition or relieve their pain. The patients then go away and improve their condition as a result of endorsing these words. The nocebo effect is when the doctor utters these words to the patient: 'Your condition will only get worse', or 'You only have three months to live'. The interpretation of these words may have devastating effects on the patient who now starts working on the process of manifesting these words. What the mind believes, it manifests. Although a blood test result show high blood sugar or high blood pressure it is up to the patient to remain on medication or seek natural therapy. There have been many cases, including my own, where alternative supplements and therapy have helped the body go back into balance again.

When we receive messages, it is the interpretations of those messages that influences our decisions in life. There are two driving forces that determines how we make these decisions. The powerful forces are LOVE and FEAR. The results we get in our life is greatly determined by our state of being during the time of the decisions; everything we think of, say, or do gets created accordingly. Needless to say that everything done through fear results in suffering, whereas when everything is done through love it is done with ease and grace. Every cell in our body resonates how we feel leaving the body to vibrate at a low or high frequency, depending on how we manage our thoughts.

Our thoughts command everything in our life. In an instant our thoughts can take us on a high – a place of total bliss, or can drag us down to a place of total darkness. In every instance we have manifested it. Everything we put out always come back to us as a boomerang. With it all comes responsibility, respect, and restoration. In life nothing is perfect as perfection is just an illusion; when we take **responsibility** for our actions, we **restore** trust, as well as **respect** within ourselves and others.

There can be no boasting, blame, or bail. **Boasting** that you are right does not cut it as it only creates negative energy in your etheric field. **Blaming** others will not erase the error but double it. **Bailing** out does not bring forgiveness, but instead allows you to give up the power of responsibility, losing respect for yourself and others, missing out on the opportunity to restore your integrity, also being whole in yourself and your life. This is how people get sick and end up with medical conditions in their lives.

We have been provided a body with its own pharmacy. The body has been designed to heal and repair itself mentally, physically, and emotionally. The body is a fascinating creation and operates efficiently as long as it is allowed to operate the way it is designed. It is our vehicle to live on this planet to assist us in completing our path whichever way we choose to.

I was not yet 30, a young mother with a small child, and at the time I was dealing with emotional, mental, and physical abuse in my marriage. I felt that I was alone and very isolated from the world. Although I had a great job, I kept to myself a lot and did not want to speak about my situation at work or socially. This created a state of mind that allowed my situation to worsen, as I did not want to divulge to my parents what I was going through. I felt quite embarrassed by my situation and put up with it for many years.

One night when it got too much I took an overdose of sleeping pills and was found by my husband when he finally got home that night. Although I was taken to the hospital and was safe, I did not realise the impact it had on my body, but most of all the impact on my child. I was on medication for a while to cope with my situation and to mask my emotional state of being. Eventually I knew that I had to get out of that prison I had enclosed myself in. I then committed to taking control of my life, getting my power back, and recreating my life anew. I finally chose not to become a victim of my circumstances. With the help of natural therapy and supplements I managed to gradually restore my health on physical, mental, and emotional level again.

This got me into a total mind shift. I applied for a new promotion and got the job. I met new people and gradually nursed myself back to health. Although I had not resolved my marital situation I was getting stronger and having more clarity on what had to be done to go to the next level in my life. I took on several activities including expanding my education and attending regular yoga sessions that helped exercise my mind, my body, and also my internal organs. It all added to the healing process. I was led to an amazing healer, coach, and mentor who helped me tap into my inner being and discover the strength within myself to feel whole again.

I eventually had the courage to face my husband and end the marriage. That time, instead of running away to a women's refuge, I made the decision to stand my ground and fearlessly took the necessary actions to detach myself emotionally, mentally, and physically from the destructive cycle that had me remain in darkness for a long time. I had seen the light and with it came the love for myself. Out of sheer bravery and enormous courage, I embraced all the encouragement and support from my coach. I became unstoppable in creating a totally new environment for myself. I did get to that place of safety and freedom. The world was unfamiliar and scary but it did not deter me from starting again. There was no certainty on where I was going or what was going to happen to me. I was ready to take on every opportunity that came my way and give it my best shot.

If you do not get in control of your thoughts then they will take control of you. I allowed this to happen for many years. My husband controlled me through my emotions which created my vulnerability. My belief and my interpretation of how a marriage should be became my reality. It kept me in a state of confusion with me clinging to what I thought could be. I lived in the future, instead of tackling the present. I thought that I could fix my life, unaware that some situations in life are beyond our control. I lived in hope even when every indication pointed towards a situation that was doomed. I thought that everything I was seeking was outside of me.

I now know that the person I should have trusted the most was ME. I was not listening to myself, but to my thoughts. How could

I have discounted seeing who I really was and how valuable I was to my life? I totally ignored my responsibility to myself and had no integrity with who I was and what was important for me, and my son. We have to be patient with our learning as it does not happen instantly. We learn to live with no judgement, even towards ourselves. It has been instrumental in building my resilience and my tenacity in not letting life beat me.

Assistance is always available. It is a matter of reaching out. "seek and you shall find", "knock and the door will be open to you." As we evolve as human beings we realise that we are not alone. I understand now how not asking brought so much suffering in my life. As a child I was always afraid of asking my father for things that I needed, as I found him unapproachable. I also felt that I was never listened to. I lived in a solitary world where nothing good existed, not even love.

Through ongoing self-development I became more confident in myself. As I made new decisions for myself I found that my thinking was changing. I gradually discovered love, faith, trust, assertiveness, and self-expression. It took a while to speak about my experiences and stop keeping my past as a secret. This has allowed feelings of freedom and reduced my alienation from the rest of the world. There was nothing to hide anymore. I no longer lived in a world of silence, or not being heard. I acquired the ability to manage fear in my life without it overtaking my whole life.

The average person processes at least 60,000 thoughts per day. We tend to be attached to nearly 95% of those thoughts, and we go through the same ones day in and day out, sometimes for months, and years. Unless we change our routine or our life dramatically we unconsciously tend to recreate the same energy pattern every single day. Each of these energy patterns then impact the body. These can be changed in an instant though. Most people are victims to society, allowing themselves to be heavily influenced by what goes on around them. We can make decisions that suit us despite what other people think. It is our life, not theirs.

The nervous system can be compared to being the body's hardware, and the chemical changes in our body that affect our thoughts, thus our emotions, can be seen as being the software. All we then need is to take the body through a de-fragmentation process to get reprogrammed again. If all this is too complicated, we then seek a specialist. In this case it will be a coach, therapist, healer, or a mentor.

Goalsetting is very much part of changing our mindset. It allows us to consider what else is possible and constantly stretch ourselves to places we have not been before. It dares us to realise dreams that we think only few people can achieve. We sometimes see some goals or dreams as being impossible, or too difficult to reach. The point of setting goals is to do things that are perceived as being impossible. You challenge yourself to go there, and celebrate when you have made 'possible' the 'impossible'. This has us discover how powerful we are as human beings. We get to experience things that make us step up and step out of our comfort zone to excel and inspire others.

Objections and responses:

When I get depressed I am unable to perform unless I take some medication.

It is fine to take medication at the onset of depression. It is even better to join a group or include some form of physical activity in your routine. Seek the advice of a therapist who can help you nurse yourself back to a healthier life and not rely on medication to live your life. In some cases it may have to be this way, but it is for you to choose how you want to live your life.

What if I cannot control my mind?

You can easily control your mind through regular meditation, coaching sessions, or other activities.

What if all this cost money?

It is easy to work out a budget to cater for our needs. We choose what is important and what is not. When we make decisions according to priority we usually get everything we want out of life.

3 actions to take as a result of reading this chapter:
1. Take risk in and expand yourself to reach the highest level in life. Feel the fear and do it anyway.
2. There are many forms of guided meditation on the internet. Practice the one that resonates with you.
3. Your self-image will always dictate your thinking and your behaviour. Be aware of it. Transform it and you will transform your life.

> 'We are what we think. All we are arises with our thoughts. With our thoughts we make the world.'
> – Buddha

Body Wisdom

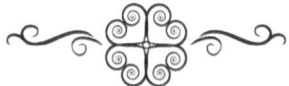

The human body has been designed to completely heal itself.

'If we are creating ourselves all the time, then it is never too late to begin creating the bodies we want instead of the ones we mistakenly assume we are stuck with.'
– Deepak Chopra

The body comes with its own repair programme. Being in tune with your body means that you can easily attend to its needs. It is your responsibility to look after your body. When we do whatever it takes to maintain and support its restoration our body loves us for it. When your body needs your attention be sure to find some time for it so it won't let you down. When you look after your body, it will look after you.

In contrast:
In the past decades we seemed to have become too reliant of medication to cure any ailments. These ailments then turned into

medical conditions. This is because medication and drugs have been heavily used. Instead of finding the cause in the first place and rectifying it, we have become used to masking our health with drugs.

When a male sex cell called the 'sperm' meets up with a female sex cell called the 'ovum' and fertilises, it becomes a zygote. The zygote then divides many times over into a cluster of cells which becomes a blastocyst. The blastocyst finally implants itself in the womb and becomes an embryo.

The human body is an incredible machine. Its intricate design works with precision allowing it to function and achieve miraculous things. The skin, being the largest organ in the human body, continually produces new cells to replace the old cells as they die. The frame, which is the skeletal system, includes all of the bone structures in the body.

The brain and the spinal cord makes up the central nervous system. The nervous system is made of billions of nerve cells. It is designed to communicate messages from the brain to the skin, organs, and other parts of the body by coordinating their functions. The nerve cells or neurons use electrical impulses to transmit information to and from different parts of the body. The communication to the neurons is transmitted via 'axons' whereas the 'dendrites' receive impulses from other parts of the body.

The cell nucleus is responsible for the basic functional unit of all tissues including the DNA which holds the genetic information about each human being. The genes are responsible for the building, maintenance, and repair of cells, and creating the unique characteristics of a person. Each individual has 100,000 genes contained in their DNA. DNA was discovered in 1953 by Francis Crick and James Watson, and stands for deoxyribonucleic acid. Also held within the cell nucleus is the mitochondrion, a very important structure that creates energy.

Amongst the specialised cells in the body are the red and white blood cells, the macrophages, the neurons, the muscle cells, and the skin cells. Each of these cells perform various functions in the body. Red blood cells develop in the bone marrow and transport oxygen and carbon dioxide via the bloodstream. The B lymphocytes and T lymphocytes in white blood cells are responsible for the immune response. Macrophages can move through the body tissues as well as travelling through the bloodstream and are responsible for defending the body against foreign materials attacking it. Muscle cells respond to hormones and nervous stimuli in the body, using electricity to perform its activities. The lymphatic or immune system is always on the alert, keeping away harmful organism and draining waste from the body. The circulatory system distributes hormones and nutrients throughout the body.

The wound healing process in the body is quite fascinating. Depending whether the wound is narrow or wide, the healing is initiated by a different process. With a narrow wound a blood clot forms in the wound, contracting then drawing the two sides of the wound together. Fibroblasts then supply a granulation tissue from the edges of the wound which is gradually replaced by the connective tissues. When the wound is open and wide it is filled with granulation tissue beginning from the base and sides of the wound until it is all filled.

From what I have researched and read the human body is constantly recreating itself at the 'quantum mechanical, atomic, and molecular level'. On a molecular level the skin cell dies and renews itself every month, and that allows the skin to be so soft and pliable. It is said that the stomach lining replaces itself every five days, the liver gets renewed every six weeks, and the skeleton gets replaced every three months. It is believed that as we breathe in oxygen the body gets renewed, and as we exhale the body gets rid of what it no longer needs. Studies also show that our DNA changes through the years of physical growth, from a baby, to adulthood, to old age. The body you have now is not the body you had last year, or the year before.

The brain is the centre of our thinking, memory, auditory, and visual association, as well as our emotions. This is where information from the special sense organs related to sight, hearing, taste, and smell gets processed. All of the vital functions are controlled by the brain. It acts as a 24-hour surveillance system that ensures the smooth operation of the whole body. The brain constantly monitors all of the body systems and functions, and alerts the responsible part of the body to respond in case of danger, damage, or injury.

There are four parts to the brain. The **cerebrum** is the largest part of the brain and is composed of white matter in the inner core and grey matter on the outer cortex. The **diencephalon** is made of two main components including the thalamus and the hypothalamus. The role of the thalamus is to relay incoming and outgoing messages between the spine and the brain. Some of these messages are then redirected to the cerebral cortex. The hypothalamus, which is located at the base of the brain, controls the autonomic nervous system, as well as monitoring temperature and hormone levels in the body. It also keeps an eye on hormone production in the pituitary gland. The **brain stem** takes care of the breathing function, the heart rate, and blood pressure in the body. It is connected to the spinal cord and acts as a relay between the spine and the brain. Finally, the **cerebellum** is attached to the brain stem. It is also referred to as the 'little brain', and is responsible for the control of movement. It coordinates the voluntary muscle activity, as well as maintaining the balance and equilibrium in the body.

The four lobes of the brain are strongly linked. The primary motor cortex of the brain is linked with the **frontal lobe**. It involves movement, thinking, behaviour, and personality, whereas the primary sensory cortex of the brain is linked with the **parietal lobe** that is involved with the perception of touch and comprehension of speech. The **occipital** and **temporal** lobes are involved with the perception of vision and memory.

Knowing that we have choices in everything that happens to us at every moment prompts us to change our thought patterns to have better results in our life. We can reprogram our mind to create anew what we do not like about ourselves, our body, or our life. We are capable of having a new body, revitalised health, and a total new life by creating those intentions NOW. Once the brain receives these intention, it starts the process promptly, sending commands throughout the body to produce the manifestation of our thoughts and desires.

It took me some time to comprehend what I am about to share with you. What I found out is that our body is made of cells. Those cells are made of molecules, which are made of atoms, and atoms are made up of subatomic particles. When there are vibrational disturbances in the body at the subatomic level it causes abnormalities at the atomic level. This then moves to the molecular level. It might take a few years before the cells get affected and then the body starts showing signs of discomfort and pain.

Since the organs are made of cells, a history of accumulation of vibrational disturbances end up as chronic diseases within the body. The organs that are governed by the endocrine system are also made of cells. This may be the reason why people in their 50s and onwards end up with conditions like diabetes, arthritis, Alzheimer's, cardiovascular diseases, and so on. These people are then prescribed medication to alleviate their conditions, but as medication helps only on a cellular level and cannot go deep to the subatomic level to heal the patient completely. These sufferers then end up on medication for the rest of their lives.

The present moment is where everything gets created. What was said and done a minute ago is already in the past. What we are thinking, creating, planning, and goalsetting now is all that will happen in the future. I am thinking now, 'It is time for me to go and make myself a smoothie'. Putting out this intention will have me get up and organise a smoothie with chia seeds. This is what I am thinking, choosing something healthy because my tummy is grumbling. So, I lock in my intention before the part of my brain that is linked with taste and memory suggests anything I remember that tastes nice like chips, biscuits, or chocolate.

I say, 'Thank you for sharing, I do remember how nice that was, but my intention is to keep lean and healthy. I am sticking to my new routine because I am conscious about what is right for my health. I know that the reward is greater if I stick with my intentions'. I am in my thought, but I am talking with myself, right? There is my ego or persona that does not care what is right for me and there is my Inner Being who knows what is right for me. I am now enjoying a blueberry smoothie with rice milk and chia seeds. It is quenching my thirst and hunger while I sip it slowly from my tall drink bottle. It is keeping my antioxidant level above 50,000 counts and my cells healthy and young. It is boosting my immune system, creating a great defence barrier from any invaders that may be lurking in my body. I am being instrumental in building what I want and what is right for me. I am committed to keep fit and healthy so I act accordingly.

The body is designed to produce chemicals that allows its smooth function. It acts like an inner pharmacy that manufactures the appropriate chemicals or drugs that repair as well as balance the body naturally, with no side-effects. Some examples are chemicals like: **serotonin**, a chemical that regulates mood, alertness, and the temperature of the body; **melatonin,** which is produced by the pineal gland and is instrumental in regulating the body clock or the circadian rhythm; and **endorphins** that soothe our pain. If the body is designed to do all of this, what is it that the body can't make to heal itself? I invite you to discover ways of healing by trusting that your body will heal itself if this is what you choose for yourself.

Objections:
I have given up on my health, I know I will never get better.
Even in acute cases people have managed to heal themselves.

I feel helpless, I have been on treatment for a long time now and my condition has not improved.

Your doctor's diagnosis will give you an indication on what is not working in the body. If you do not improve with treatment, do your own research and get additional advice or a second opinion.

Apart from doctors, who else can I get a second opinions from?

There are lots of therapists out there. Start with a naturopath at your local health food store. Ask as many questions as you can to get the answer that you want. Go with what you feel is right for you.

3 actions to take as a result of reading this chapter:

1. If you are suffering from any conditions, ask for advice and seek for answers until you find the right treatment for yourself.
2. Be in awe of the function of the human body and what it is capable of. Educate yourself in a way that you discover the miracle of the human body and life itself.
3. Discover the secret of healing and you will be astounded by the miracles it can produce in your life.

> 'The body is ... a field of simultaneity where physics, chemistry, biology and mathematics all come together.'
> – Deepak Chopra

Our Beliefs

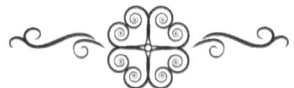

Your beliefs may not be yours but you will learn from them.

'When you want something, all the universe
conspires in helping you to achieve it.'
– Paulo Coelho

Your beliefs stem from how you were raised and how you have been conditioned to them as you grew up. We are brought up with belief systems and traditions. As we grow up we observe our parents and believe what they believe. As we observe people around us, what becomes apparent is that children who are brought up in a safe environment and surrounded by love tend to excel in their lives. Those who have been brought up by parents who have not contributed to them seem to struggle. The world is made of light and darkness; some fall into the light and others totally fall into the darkness.

The world is full of suffering, and it is difficult to comprehend why this is so. Many human beings spend their lives contributing to healing the world so there is less suffering. Even for those who succeed in life, we find that at some point they have to go through challenges to reach enlightenment just like the rest of us. There is so much learning for all human beings and it is a blessing when great teachers appear in our lives. Nevertheless, we are meant to learn from each other. After all, we are all connected. When we learn to accept ourselves for who we are and accept those around us, life becomes easier and more peaceful.

Many people have become successful despite a very poor or traumatic upbringing by modelling their heroes, someone who inspires them. This is the way they turn their life around and end up achieving great things. They manage to find that burning flame that gives them the desire to pursue their dreams. They learn to tap into the abundance that already exist around them and find the prosperity that the Universe provides for us all.

Another form of attachment that brings so much pain and suffering in the world is religion. Looking at the main religions of the world we find a lot of history and traditions. All religions come from the Middle East and Asia. Jerusalem is considered to be holy for the three monotheistic religions: Judaism, Christianity, and Islam.

Sadly, since the classical times until today there is still conflict between Israel and Palestine over the city of Jerusalem. The Temple of Solomon has great significance for all three religions because it is believed that it is the site where Abraham, the prophet sacrificed his son. Although today, many are turning back to the philosophy of the ancient religions of the East such as Hinduism and Buddhism.

Religion is meant to be a guide to stay spiritually connected to God, our Creator. It has us aligned with our virtues and moral values. It has us respect other human beings and everything that is sacred on this planet. We turn to religion to keep us connected to the essence of who we really are and to nourish our souls through prayers so we do not lose our way. The 10 Commandments are the laws that were handed to Moses to give us a clear guideline for human beings; honour each other and respect and preserve life on this planet.

Throughout the centuries, there have been many teachers, sages and prophets, who have been sent to us to create a peaceful world: Abraham, Moses, Buddha, Jesus the Son of God, Muhammad, and others. Each time we were sent a prophet a new religion was born, and there has been a holy book to follow. Each Holy Book comes with different messages to address the evolution of men on this planet. As humanity evolves, we receive messages on a higher level.

It is believed that Gautama Buddha, the Enlightened One, and founder of Buddhism, lived approximately between 560 – 480BC. At the age of 29 he went through a radical change in his life. After severe fasting he realised that he was not on the right path. He eventually sat under a Bodhi tree and meditated for four weeks until he reached enlightenment. He then recruited five disciples and started the 'Wheel of Teaching'. He understood that life was connected to suffering and his teachings were about how to overcome suffering.

Part of the teachings of Buddha is observing 'The Four Noble Truths':

1. There is suffering.
2. Suffering has a cause: craving.
3. If craving ceases, suffering ceases.
4. There is a path leading to the cessation of suffering. The Eightfold Path is the answer to the end of suffering and comprises of three divisions: Wisdom, Moral Conduct, and Control of Mind.

Buddha passed into nirvana at the age of 80.

As in early Christianity, Gautama Buddha's teachings were recorded by his disciples and followers. As authorised by U Ba Khin, the teachings of Gautama Buddha continue at the various Vipassana Meditation Centres around the world. There are six centres in Australia that offer 10-day meditation courses, as well as 20, 30, and 90-day ones. I attended my first 10-day course in Queensland in July this year which was a totally transformational experience.

The Christian Church was formed after the Pentecost experience of the apostles. Paul, originally Saul, one of Jesus' apostles formulated the main principles of Christianity and the faith in Jesus Christ. In Christianity, Jesus Christ came to earth as the Son of God and Son of Man. His message to humanity was to love one another. Jesus asked that humanity renounce power and violence. Jesus was arrested in Jerusalem and was crucified at the age of 33 with the approval of Pontius Pilate.

The main scriptures of Catholicism are compiled in *The Holy Bible*. It includes the Old Testament, New Testament, and the gospels of Mathew, Mark, Luke, and John, among other scriptures and writings.

As it has been narrated in many history books. At age 40, Muhamad was visited in a dream by the angel Gabriel who commanded him to read a book, and told him that he was a prophet of God. Muhammad, founder of Islam, started preaching in Mecca in 610AD. It was said that Muhammad and his followers were being ridiculed and becoming a victim of campaigns from the rich citizens of Mecca. They comprised Arabs, Jewish, and Christians of Mecca. He was banished to Medina in 622, and in 630 Muhammad took arms against his home town of Mecca. He then made the Ka'aba into a purely Muslim shrine, built in honour of the prophet Abraham and monotheism. People from the Muslim faith believe Allah to be the only God and Muhammad to be the last prophet. The holy book of Islam is the *Koran*.

Jewish people believe that Yahveh is the one and only God, and one of God's names is the 'Eternal' (Isaiah 44:6). A system of reward and punishment where God or Yahveh is the judge was devised by Judaism and later adopted by Christianity, and also Islam. Followers of Judaism believe that the Torah is God's law and it is all contained in The Five Books of Moses, or the Pentateuch.

It is said that the Jewish calendar started with the creation of the world. The Christian year 1240 corresponds to the Jewish year 5000.

Kabbalah is a term used since the 13th century for Jewish mysticism. Author Tim Dedopulos refers to it as 'God's blueprint for creation or the key to unlocking your ultimate potential'; kabbalah meaning 'to receive' or 'to accept' offers a wealth or wisdom. It also contains specific techniques for improving the mind, body, and soul. In other words, it helps shed light on the process of the creation of the Universe and the purpose of life on Earth.

The Tree of Life—The Otz Chiim

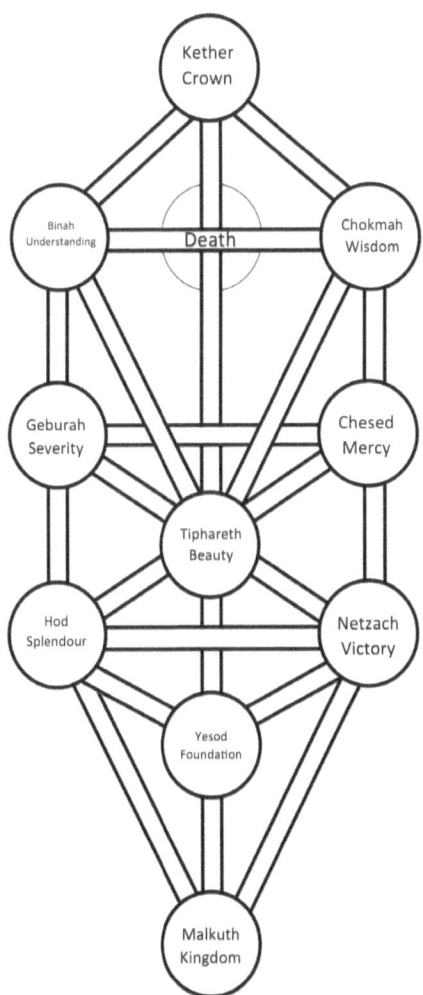

The Path to Self-Perfection
The Sacred Centre of Kabbalistic Teaching

Kether – Crown	**Kether** meaning the 'Crown'- source of the Divine, the great 'I AM'
	Associated with the planet Pluto as well as the consciousness, diamond, the almond scent, lotuses, the almond trees, swans ...
Binah & Chokmah (Understanding & Wisdom)	**Binah** meaning 'Understanding' also known as 'Marah' – the great sea.
	Associated with the planet Saturn as well as the right side of the brain, pearl, myrrh, lilies, birch trees, chalices, sirens, whales ...
	Chokmah meaning 'Wisdom' or intelligence also referred as the Holy Father or the word of God.
	Associated with the planet Neptune as well as Left side of the brain, the gemstone turquoise, frankincense, orchids, beech trees, owls ...
Geburah & Chesed (Severity & Mercy)	**Geburah** meaning 'Severity' which can be translated as strength, might and power.
	Also known as 'Din' – law or 'Pakhad' -fear
	Associated with the planet Mars as well as the adrenal glands, the gemstone ruby, cypress, peonies, rowan trees, swords, spears, horses ...
	Chesed meaning 'Mercy' which denotes compassion and loving kindness
	Associated with the planet Jupiter as well as the shoulders, the gemstone sapphire, cedarwood, tulips, crop fields, birch trees, sphinxes, dolphins ...
Tiphareth – Beauty	**Tiphareth** meaning 'Beauty' and harmony. Also known as 'Rokhmim' or mercy
	Associated with the sun as well as home, the heart, the gemstone topaz, rose, holly trees, spiders ...
Hod & Netzach (Splendour & Victory)	**Hod** meaning 'Glory' and translated as splendour, majesty, brightness and beauty.
	Associated with the planet mercury as well as the kidney, the gemstone Fire Opal, rosemary, pansies, hazel trees, foxes ...
	Netzach meaning 'Victory' and translated as endurance, faithfulness, permanence, eternity, excellence, completion and perfection.
	Associated with the planet venus as well as the Solar Plexus, the gemstone emerald, patchouli, apple tree, the dove ...
Yesod – Foundation	**Yesod** meaning 'Foundation' also known as 'Tzaddik', meaning righteousness
	Associated with the moon as well as the sexual organs, lavender, violet, willow trees, incence, mirrors, cats ...
Malkuth – Kingdom	**Malkuth** - Base of the 'Tree of Life' also known as 'Shekhinah'- refers to the female aspect of God. It represents the state of being.
	Associated with Mother Earth - cradle of our life as well as the human body, the gemstone rock crystal, sandalwood, clover, oak trees, rabbits ...

Hinduism spread rapidly during the Classical Period, around 500BC. At the time Sanskrit (an artificial language of poet and scholars) was used for religious purposes. Around 1000BC the Vedic Sanskrit speakers, Aryans, advanced east and south of Punjab to the Ganges and introduced the caste system. The new gods were then Brahma, Vishnu, and Shiva. The most important Hindu texts are the four Vedas, the associated Brahmana, and the Upanishads.

We are attached to our views and beliefs, convinced that they are the only one that counts. It seems to be the same with traditions; we carry on the traditions we are used to, until there comes a point when we have to give them up, to evolve and go to the next level in life. As I watched a documentary on Diana, Princess of Wales, I saw how she was instrumental in changing the tradition of the Royal Family. Even though she was not born a royal, the people of England demanded that she receive a royal state funeral. Diana was devoted to them through her dedicated duties to the monarchy.

Our senses are conditioned to see the world a certain way, when in reality it is beyond our comprehension. It was once believed that the Earth was flat, until it was discovered to be round. We perceived this planet to be stationary in space, yet science tells us that the Earth is spinning on its own axis at thousands of miles an hour.

We are now learning the ancient religion or spiritual philosophy of how the Universe works, and our role in it. We sometimes do not have the whole answer, but we are getting on the path to peace for all of humanity, because that is what God wants for us.

Objections and responses:

Is it important to be religious?

Some religions claim to be better than the others. Jesus Christ said, 'Love one another, like my father loves you'. If we are divided and cannot love each other, no religion can ever take us to enlightenment and be closer to God, Our Creator.

I believe what my parents believe, that's ok with me.

That is fine. As long as you believe in something that has you value yourself and everyone around you and gives you a sense of purpose in life.

I don't know who to trust. Religion is confusing. My parents are from different religions.

Trust in yourself. All that you need to know is that you have the answer all inside you. Follow the religion that suits you. We are all praying to the same God, our Creator.

3 actions to take as a result of reading this chapter:
1. We are not here to accept what we are being told anymore. This is a concept of the past where we were fed information that we end up believing. With technology we now have access to an abundance of resources and information. This is the way to discover your own truth.
2. Pursue a life that brings you fulfilment guided by virtues that nourish your life and your soul.
3. We seem to be here, not only for ourselves but also for the good of the whole planet. Seek the transformation you need and you will be guided to transform the whole world.

> 'The only person you are destined to become is the person you decide to become.'
> – Ralph Waldo Emerson

Beyond Medication

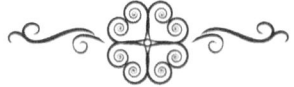

*Natural remedies and supplements heal the body
faster and with no side effects.*

'To keep the body in good health is a duty …
otherwise we shall not be able to keep our
mind strong and clear.'
– Buddha

When we are prescribed medication as a result of some ailment, we can consider this as a short-term remedy, giving time for the body to retrain itself and recover. We must be aware that being on medication for long-term prevents the body from correcting itself. The idea is to start researching what diagnosis was received and track down which part of the body is not functioning well. This will help us find out which supplement or therapy can be implemented to gently nurse the body into the right rhythm again. When transitioning from medical prescriptions to a natural supplement or remedy it is best done under the supervision of a naturopath or someone qualified. Some diseases or sicknesses may stem from an imbalance on an emotional or psychological level and can be corrected.

Research has shown that the body is able to renew its organs and even its skeletal muscle. It is believed that through yoga practice and meditation that the coronary arteries can be cleared of 'fatty acid plaques' completely. Added to these practices a modified diet can be introduced to eliminate permanent medical prescriptions and surgery procedures.

In contrast:
Receiving bad news from a diagnosis can lead people to give up on themselves. Some will allow their health to deteriorate even further. Some cannot commit to the restoration of their health and get resigned to permanently be on medication. It seems to be the easier way out as it becomes too hard to find a better solution.

When we encounter serious illness we may feel totally helpless. We become confused and afraid. Once in that state of mind it is difficult to act rationally. When the immune system is down we lose our focus and our energy plummets to a very low vibration. It all gets too difficult to handle, so we are then willing to hand over the decision to someone else. Most of the time it is the medical professionals that we rely on because we think that they are the only ones who have studied how the human body functions. We therefore expect them to have the right answer for our ailments. We know how poor we are feeling but cannot fathom what has gone wrong, and whether we contributed to the situation. We even get to lose faith in ourselves.

Childhood illness is something we all have to grow up with. Vaccination has helped minimise deaths and the adverse symptoms of sufferers for centuries. Without the implementation of vaccines there would have been devastation such as the plague that killed 1.5 million people in England between 1348 and 1350. Third-world countries are in need of vaccination because they are still affected by poor hygiene and sanitation. Vaccination has led to the eradication of polio around the world and to date there are only a few cases left in two countries, Afghanistan and Pakistan. Rotary International, backed by Bill Gates, have been instrumental in this successful campaign.

We are very grateful for Louis Pasteur's contribution to science, technology, and medicine in the 1800s. The French chemist and microbiologist discovered that microorganisms caused fermentation and disease. He also developed vaccines against anthrax and rabies. He saved so many lives, and helped countless others. All his medical research and discoveries are still being applied in hospital and clinics to help humans and animals today.

These days, some parents are totally against vaccinating their children. Some medical conditions that children suffer in our day and age can be managed without vaccines. Children suffering from asthma, eczema, and certain viruses can be remedied with natural therapy, essential oils, or a modified diet.

Living in advanced countries such as Australia and America, we do not have to deal with malnutrition but instead with overeating and the consumption of high fats and sugars through our food intake. Once upon a time, the people affected by diabetes were between 50-60 years of age, now small children are being affected by this disease. Most of them have to resort to insulin injections. While some of the older generations are staying healthier and younger, today small children are now being affected by diseases that once affected older people. Cancer is one of them.

Louise Hay's *You Can Heal Your Life* have a lot of explanation and answers to different chronic conditions that affect us. When we are affected by a certain condition it is important to seek an answer from within – we cannot discount the medical institution all together as it is part of science and progress. It is a relief to know that organ transplants such as a new heart can give someone a new lease on life. When the body is damaged and cannot be reversed naturally, the medical world provides some amazing solution for people to resume a normal life. Medical science has produced some amazing procedures that are extending peoples' lives, or give them access to marginal improvement in their everyday life. Accidents or injuries that have impacted the use of limbs have been repaired or replaced successfully. Science plays a huge part in finding new cures and new ways to repair the human body.

Through sensation, perception, cognition, and reaction of mind and body we experience suffering at a deeper level. Some people get attached to their sickness or disease and identify themselves as that. Others will allow themselves to get sick or worsen their medical condition by indulging on drugs or medication. Someone once shared with me that he had a couple of slipped discs in his back. I shared with him how I was able to heal myself in a short time from the same ailment. He admitted to not wanting to heal because he enjoyed taking the prescription drugs He admitted to not wanting to heal because he enjoyed taking the prescription drugs.

When I was first diagnosed with diabetes in 2015 I was shocked, but at the same time I realised that I had pushed my body too far. I had committed to a project that was taking me away from having a good restful sleep to replenish my body. I was not nourishing my body the way I was meant to. I was not being responsible for my health.

I ignored the fact that I had a lot of pressure put on me from people who did not appreciate my health and what I was going through. I waited until my body gave up on me completely before I stood up and took action. I had let myself down and could not blame anyone else but myself, because no one is responsible for my wellbeing except me.

That turned out to be a big lesson for me, but it was also a big test on how I was going to remedy the situation. It shows that stress plus the lack of taking care of the body can have dire consequences resulting in illness and physical suffering. By defying the odds we can create a new paradigm shift that can create total healing. It shows that having the sheer determination to reclaim your health back and making the right decision as well as committing to it can produce massive results.

I knew I had to repair my body because I was responsible for damaging it. I did not know how I was to going to go about it but I was willing to do whatever was needed to achieve it. Once the decision was made everything got easy. I found the right therapist, the right supplements, the right regime, and the right mindset to make it all happen.

I took it on with a lot of dedication, love, and patience. I knew my body needed my attention, so I gave it all it needed in the form of exercise, breathing correctly, meditation, and more. I avoided anything that did not contribute to it. I nurtured and nourished my body with the best food and fruits and what was beneficial to my skin, my endocrine system, hair, limbs, and all my senses.

Guess what? I did it. After one year of my regime and carefully attending to my health I lost 10kg and have never felt better. I was able to stop all medications with a few months of the diagnosis. I got an antioxidant scan that confirmed that my Skin Carotenoid Score had gone up to 65,000 counts. This gave me the biggest boost ever as I knew that it was all possible. With that trust and belief I was able to create some outstanding results. So, I am now convinced that anything you believe can be achieved.

Objections and responses:

When I get ill, I feel paralysed and do not know what to do.
Once you have accepted the disease, you can start working towards letting it go.

I inherited my medical condition because of my parents. There is nothing I can do about it.
You think that you have no choice because these health conditions have been passed onto you through your genes. It has been proven that you can change your gene's expression. There are products and supplements readily available on the market to achieve that.

There are also machines available to measure and show the results.

I have to accept the doctor's diagnosis because they are the expert.

You need to go to your GP to do the required tests and monitor your health, especially if you are not confident on what is the next step to take. You can choose to take prescribed medication or not. You have to choose a responsible way to restore your health guided by someone who has the knowledge unless you have acquired it yourself.

3 actions to take as a result of reading this chapter:
1. Avoid being stuck in fear, and overwhelmed. Feel it all, then open your toolbox and start the repair process.
1. Keep asking questions until you find the right cure or therapist who will guide you on your journey of self-healing.
2. Make sure you give your body all the attention it needs to repair any damage and produce a full recovery. Usually when we fall sick, it is a wakeup call to start looking at our health and start restoring it. It is usually an initial warning that something is not right in the body.

> 'The first wealth is health.'
> – Ralph Waldo Emerson

Food Essence

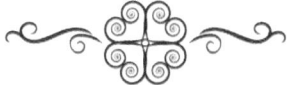

Our body needs wholesome food and wholesome management.

'Let food be thy medicine and medicine be thy food.'
– Hippocrates

The body is a sacred gift; it should be nurtured and appreciated. You cannot accept any food that is given to you without asking yourself, 'Is this the right food for my body?' When you live in a culture that allows you to eat at restaurants more often than at home, you have to be mindful that the food you order is a healthy choice. Depending on your body type, your weight, and health status you are responsible for choosing the appropriate meal each day to serve your body. You should ask yourself, 'Does my body need lots of food today, or less food?' We must eat according to the daily requirement of our body. Overeating as much as undereating can be harmful to the body. A very important reminder is to chew your food so it is processed effectively and without putting any stress on your organs.

Apart from a healthy breakfast, one large meal per day is quite sufficient and ideally consumed around lunchtime, with a light dinner to follow. Depending on your physical activities, the size of your meal may vary accordingly. Some blood types may include meat in their diet, especially those who are physically active. Depending on how the animals are fed, and slaughtered. There are reports that a lot of animals have chemicals such as hormones injected in them. Whatever the animals have gone through, when you eat that meat it is said that it gets to affect your health. These days many men as well as women choose a vegetarian diet and eat organically.

As we go back to basics we find that there is an abundance of food in the world. Brown rice and legumes can be inexpensive and healthy for your body. Legumes cooked with spices, accompanied with salads and fresh herbs make delicious and nutritious meals. Brown rice is a complete food in itself and you do not need to eat a lot as it keeps your stomach full longer and digested very slowly by the body. It contains protein and fat, as well as calcium, magnesium, silicium, phosphorous, vitamins, and minerals.

To manage your weight it may be beneficial to get into a routine of adding frozen berries to some protein powder (pea and brown rice, preferably) to make a smoothie. Coconut and rice milk is a good alternative to cow's milk and is available in coffee shops. When going for a meeting, instead of having a coffee which can become addictive, especially the non-organic ones, you may choose a much healthier choice of Earl Grey tea, Chai tea, or even a turmeric latte (made from coconut milk) – usually available in coffee shops.

Berries are very high in antioxidants and are great to add to smoothies. A long drink can be a berry or green drink in a tall drink bottle with a couple of dessert spoons of chia seeds added. It provides great nutrition value and keeps your stomach full. The added benefit is that it leaves less room for those expensive snacks that you do not need to fill your body with. Most of them are full of sugar, too much salt, and added chemicals that will not serve your body.

The fact shows that during WWII the Queensland Government was concerned that rationing people on the home front would result in the deterioration of their health; in fact it helped reduce the health issues like obesity, heart disease, and diabetes.

In contrast:
Most people eat foods that are heavily processed. This interferes with the normal body functions and its rejuvenation, and can cause inflammation. Most of the common conditions like arthritis, diabetes, and fibromyalgia are caused by inflammation in the body. Some genetically modified foods can have adverse effects on one's health, so choose your food carefully. There are inexpensive food like pulses or legumes that can be stored and cooked anytime. It usually requires longer cooking time but who does not have a crockpot that can produce excellent meals especially for winter nights. Even if you live in an apartment in the city, you can still grow herbs and some salads on the balcony. It is easy to create a semi-shade area to assist any plant to grow healthy. Organic food are healthier and keeps longer. Quality sourced food will offer you vitality and longevity.

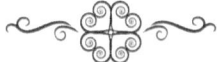

As we advance in age our body function slows down. In fact, it actually starts to degenerate. We have to be conscious on how to maintain our vitality and wellbeing. We tend to take things for granted until it is too late. Unless we have health-conscious parents or are influenced by people who value their health, we tend to eat anything. Most of the time we eat anything that is put in front of us, not even considering whether it will nourish our body or not. If it is tasty and fills the hole in our stomach we seem to be happy with it, especially when we do not have to cook for ourselves.. This is why companies like McDonald's and many others have such profitable businesses. Ideally, we should have some raw food as well as some cooked food in our diet every day. Some foods have more nutrition when eaten raw or lightly steamed, especially if it is organically grown.

I was raised in a large family of nine people where my father was the only breadwinner. Our meals were limited, but mum was always creative, using lots of legumes or pulses, adding raw and cooked vegetables to our meals; we consumed very little meat or fish. I suppose that my father could not afford it, so we would have meat and fish on special occasions. I do remember eating dried fish and salted meat occasionally.

Since my early twenties I have been health-conscious. I worked with a colleague who introduced me to the Zen Macrobiotic philosophy. She also got me interested in vitamins and supplements and suggested certain books that were very valuable reading. I still have these books in my library, and they have made this book possible. I got to understand how to use vitamin supplements to prevent, manage, and reverse any illness, and generally to improve my health and keep my stamina. As a working mum I could not afford to take time off work, so every autumn I devised a course of vitamins for myself and my son to boost our immune system. When winter came we would sometimes have a mild cold and had the ability to shake it off quickly and with hardly any symptoms.

When I arrived in Australia more than 40 years ago I weighed only six stone. I had lost so much weight from being seasick while travelling on a Greek ship to reach the Australian shores. Growing up, my eldest sister would constantly make fun of me. I felt so bad about the way I looked then. I was always envious of her and her girlfriends who had curves, whereby I had none. Today, being skinny is quite the way to go. Who would have thought that things would change so much? As people's mindset changes, everything changes.

I arrived on the Gold Coast in 2004 and, being in a new relationship, lived a life of abundance. I was eating what I thought was the best for me; huge meals at restaurants, as well as indulging in lots of wine, spirits, and liqueurs. I was not aware at the time that I was putting my body through so much hard work. Never did I think that I would have any health issues. Everything in moderation allows us to enjoy the experience with added benefits.

In 2013 I was diagnosed with Type II diabetes. I was on prescribed medication from my GP. My two eldest sisters were also diabetic sufferers. They had been on medication for quite some years and had also been treated with insulin injections. Initially I felt overwhelmed and petrified. They were convinced that due to the fact that my mother suffered from high cholesterol and diabetes that they had no choice but to accept their predicament. Whenever I visited the doctors in the past they would always ask if anyone in the family had any of these conditions. They would then imply that it was hereditary and that I would end up becoming a victim as well. When I shared my plight with my sisters, they were ready to welcome me in their 'camp'. I decided otherwise and declined their invitation. I knew that I did not have to take on this condition. We all have choices and I took up the freedom to choose what I wanted for myself. Mind you, I had no idea how I was going to heal myself but I knew I could do it. I had defied the odds in the past with great results. I had this inner knowing that all was well and that I had to trust my intuition all the way.

Once I made the decision, everything came my way. It all unfolded, and it was as if the doors were opening to me one by one. It became an amazing journey. I took control of my health again. Based on my past experiences I worked out a list of supplements with guidance from a few nutritionists. I also read avidly on the subject as well as watching videos and doing other research. I urgently reviewed my diet and got rid of all bread, cakes, biscuits, and all packaged food, including snacks, and even cereals.

I took up walking, making it the first thing I attended to every morning. I only drank water prior to the walk to burn the fat that I had in storage. Fruit was the first thing I ate in the morning. I was committed to a low-sugar fruits regime such as green apples, strawberries, etc., and rigidly followed a blood type diet that I'd started a few years prior. This actually gave me a basis to start with. Should you have the same condition you may be able come up with a different healing process that would suit you best. This is my experience and may not apply to anyone else. When we are in tune with our body the right treatment will always come our way as long as we seek it.

Within two months I was able to stop my medication and take some supplements instead. The main goal was to keep my sugar level balanced and reduce my weight. When attending parties and eating at restaurants I find that the blood type diet helps me stick to the right food. Since I had stopped drinking alcohol, it became a blessing in getting rid of the excess chemicals and sugars that these drinks contain. It allowed me to restore my health much faster than I anticipated.

Today I avoid consuming wheat-base products such as packaged cereals, toast, crumpets, and pancakes. I stick to brown rice, black rice, wild rice, basmati rice, and often have quinoa cooked with some turmeric (good for inflammation, since diabetes is an inflammation disease). My smoothies are made of frozen berries, rice or coconut milk, water, and brown rice and pea protein. The evening meal is a small portion of meat or fish with three or four serves of vegetables, mostly greens. I regularly have a gentle liver detox. Chromium and cinnamon bark are excellent for sugar balance. I believe CoQ10 helps in renewing the mitochondria in our cells. Meditation calms and re-centres the body, whereas regular walks or yoga or any form or physical exercise helps with oxygenating the body and renewing our cells.

It is believed that the American government used ammonium nitrate and poisonous gas left after the war to produce fertilisers and pesticides. The agricultural industry benefited hugely from subsidised fertilisers from the government. Financial incentive saw the farming of corn and soy being produced in large quantities. This was then added to packed food to produce long shelf-life and inexpensive food to feed the mass population after the war.

We have pretty much followed America's footsteps in endorsing manufactured products high in fructose corn syrup, hydrogenated oil, and modified corn starches and soy. All these products are readily available on our supermarket shelves wherever we go. All the available snacks and soft drinks are saturated with sugar and chemicals, poisoning our body and disrupting the orderly flow of our body mechanism.

As we are being awakened we become aware how our food supply as well as our water supply get laced with all sorts of chemicals that we cannot even pronounce. There are many systems available to alkalise or purify your water system. Our body is approximately 70% water, which is why is it important to have chemical-free water to not only quench our thirst, but also keep our body hydrated and healthy.

Objections and responses:

I don't like cooking.

Soups are easy to prepare and can be frozen for cooking-free nights. Keep plenty of frozen berries in the freezer for smoothies. Keep some cooked quinoa in the fridge or freezer and you will have something wholesome to eat even when you do not feel like cooking.

I always have vegetables perishing in the crisper before I get to cook them.

Take the time to purchase your produce from the organic fruit markets. You might end up spending a little more money, but organic products last much longer. When buying in bulk, share with someone or make meals that can go in the freezer for the non-cooking nights.

I love eating meat. I cannot be a vegetarian.

People of the O-type blood group are said to be meat-eaters, as this was the original blood type. It is best to eat meat from animals that have been killed in a humane way so there are no toxins remaining in the flesh. I believe that halal meat goes through a rigid process that makes it holy and is healthier for your body. Some people from the O-type group have shared with me that they do not like meat and prefer vegetarianism. It definitely is a choice.

3 actions to take as a result of reading this chapter:
1. Intentionally eliminate all packaged food from your diet and replace them with healthier snacks like fruit, nuts, and even raw or blanched vegetables.
2. Eliminate all sugars, especially white sugar (poison). Consuming natural sugars in all fresh raw food is better for the body.
3. Eliminate white flour (contains no goodness) completely from your diet. Replace with spelt and other flours – coconut, chick pea, etc.

> 'Food brings people together on many different levels. It's nourishment of the soul and body; it's truly love.'
> – Giada De Laurentiis

Tasty and Wholesome

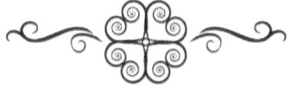

*Joyful food that not only nourishes
but also tastes great.*

'A recipe has no soul. You, as the cook, must
bring soul to the recipe.'
– Thomas Keller

Buying from the local organic market has you more connected with the food that you are going to eat. When purchasing organic vegetables we find that they taste better and keep fresher much longer. In supermarkets the vegetables may have been subject to transportation and are not as fresh. Some fruit may be out of season and have been stored for quite some time before you purchase them. The farmers may have used a lot of pesticides to produce them for the big supermarket stores.

There are more places now where you can purchase organic vegetables and fruits, including Coles and Woolworths stores. When taking your fresh purchase home, organise yourself to eat the most perishable items first. In winter this is the time to chop the vegetables and cook a nutritious soup to store in the freezer for a quick hearty meal to come home to.

Are the vegetables going be steamed, blanched, or served raw? What type of sauce are we going to serve with them; a freshly-made tomato sauce accompanied with mushroom and capsicum, or a béchamel or white sauce made from spelt flour and rice milk? How about a beautiful pumpkin sauce cooked with onion and nicely chopped mushroom to serve with some freshly cooked large size ravioli, filled with ricotta cheese and spinach? Yum!

Fruits like peaches, pears, and plums can be stewed and served with oats or brown rice for a healthy breakfast. To sweeten and spice your stewed fruit add some agave and cinnamon bark while cooking. Cinnamon is excellent for diabetic sufferers as it helps balance the sugar level in the body.

Chia is one of the highest plant-based sources of complete **protein**. It can stay fresh, ready to eat for a period of two years without preservative. It is sugar-free, gluten-free and contains a high level of antioxidant. It has 15 times more magnesium than Broccoli, eight times more Omega 3 than salmon, six times more Omega 3 than salmon, six times more **antioxidants** than blueberries, six times more **calcium** than whole milk, and three times more **iron** than spinach.

Ancient grains, pulses, or legumes can be served at any time. It is great for your main meal of the day accompanied with a hot or cold salad, salsa, and other raw side dishes. They are great to add to vegetable soups, just let them cook for at least one hour or two. Pulses or legumes are quite good if a family have a low food budget. Cover with boiled water and soak for one hour, prior to cooking. Drain before adding to pan. It speeds up the cooking process. Apart from that they are packed with vitamins and have high nutrition value.

Most foods are easy to prepare, so the simpler the better. For fresh vegetables, minimum cooking is required to lock in the goodness and preserve all the flavour. Mixing colourful vegetables makes them appealing to the eyes and inviting to the palate. Leafy greens need very little cooking and are perfect just steamed, or added raw to smoothies. When preparing salads it is great to include colours and textures providing a combination of taste. Add a drizzle of olive oil and a good squeeze of lemon or lime juice, including salt and pepper. Greens like beetroot top can be cooked in some garlic and ginger and provide some nutritious meals, and served with rice. Nothing gets discarded.

Fruits provide a great variety of vitamins, minerals, and fibre to the body. It is said that as the fruit is mixed with the saliva through the chewing process it readily turns alkaline. It may be a good idea to check with your blood type to see which fruit works best for you. This is very important for the diabetic sufferers considering some fruits contain more sugar than others.

Living in tropical regions invites anyone to eat raw. It is recommended to eat home-grown food or food that has been grown in the same region.

I was born in Mauritius, which has a diverse culture of Indian, Chinese, Creoles from Africa and Madagascar. The island was once a French colony. My cooking style is heavily influenced by French and Asian cooking but I love cooking a good Mauritian curry.

Chokos are usually regarded as a boring and bland vegetables. I was brought up on chokos, and love this vegetable so much. It must be eaten as soon as it is picked from the vine. When bought from the shop it has often been refrigerated for too long, so it has no taste. Apparently during the Depression years in Australia it was used as a jam filler. It is a native of Mexico but in other countries it has different names such as chayote, christophine, pear squash, or chu chu. In Mauritius it was known as chou chou. It provides potassium, Vitamin C, iron, magnesium, and B6. The rumour is that McDonald's used it in their apple pie. If this is so, you are still getting some nutrition value in your food.

Choko in Béchamel Sauce
- 2 chokos
- 2tb spelt flour
- Ghee, butter, or olive oil
- 1 small brown onion, sliced
- Fresh parsley
- Grated parmesan cheese

Place chokos in a pan and cover with water. Bring to boil. Simmer until cooked. Remove from pan, saving the liquid, and peel or remove skin with knife when cool. Cut in half if desired.

In a pan place either some ghee, butter, or olive oil, or combine olive oil and butter. Brown sliced onion, add the spelt flour and mix constantly. Allow to brown until it looks like breadcrumbs. Add half cup of liquid from cooked chokos. Stir briskly so it does not form lumps. Add half cup of milk of your choice to make a nice white sauce. Blend in parmesan and sprinkle with chopped parsley.

Return peeled chokos back to pan. Reheat and serve with any meat or fish or your choice or on its own. It could go well with a small piece of eye or scotch fillet. If you are a vegetarian serve with a tomato or avocado salsa using chopped fresh tomatoes, coriander, and red onion, and flavour with a few drops of sesame oil, olive oil, and salt and pepper.

Yellow split peas and chokos
- ½ cup/1 cup of yellow split peas (soaked in boiled water for 30 minutes, then repeat the process again)
- 1 large brown onion, diced
- 1 clove of garlic crushed with salt
- 1 to 2 tsp or curry powder (1 hot and 1 mild)
- 1 to 2 large chokos (with gloves on) or while soaking in a bowl of water, cut in half and peeled, then cut again into four pieces – remove the small part in the centre as it gets stringy after cooking

Pour ghee or olive oil in a pan. Gently sauté onion and garlic. Add curry powder and mix well. Add soaked and drained yellow split peas to pan. Mix well then add choko pieces. Add 4 to 6 cups of boiling water. Add 1 teaspoon of Himalayan salt or sea salt. Mix well. Bring to the boil and then cook on medium heat for one hour. Add water if necessary.

Serve with brown rice, wild rice, or basmati rice, accompanied with a garden salad with lemon and olive oil dressing.

Choko Preserve
- 2 or 3 chokos
- One large brown onion, chopped
- 1 or 2 cloves of garlic
- 1 tsp of turmeric
- ½ tsp mustard powder
- 2 to 3 tbsp of cider vinegar

Peel and grate chokos (use glove as there is a sticky gel that comes out once cut). Sprinkle with sea salt and let stand. After 10 minutes, squeeze and place on tea towel and place in the sun to dry for two hours, or dry in slow oven for about 20 minutes. When dry enough, heat oil in a wok or deep frying pan until fairly hot. Toss in the chopped onion, garlic, and turmeric. Mix well, allowing moisture to evaporate from onion and garlic mixture.

Toss in the chokos and mix well. Cook for a further five minutes then turn off the stove. Add two tablespoons of vinegar and let stand until cooled. Sterilise jars and fill with preserve after completely cooled. Keep in fridge and serve with any rice dish or quinoa.

Green mangoes, bitter lemon, or a combination or finely chopped vegetables like carrot, cabbage, green beans, and cauliflower can be preserved the same way. Some people like to add chilli as well. Turmeric is extremely good for any inflammation disease like diabetes or Arthritis. No chilli should be added if you suffer from any of an inflammation disease.

Turmeric Brown Rice Porridge

This porridge is immune-boosting, anti-inflammatory, warming, soothing, and healing.

- Organic brown rice, cooked.
- Organic rice milk
- Turmeric powder
- Cardamom
- Cinnamon
- Fennel seeds

Mix well. Heat up and serve.

Although this is not my recipe, I am sharing it because this can be used as a remedy for those suffering from, diabetes, fibromyalgia and arthritis.

Yellow Quinoa

- ½ cup quinoa
- 1 cup of boiled water

Add 1 tsp of turmeric (to alternate the flavour add 1/4 tsp of ground cumin or caraway seed)

Add a few drops of olive oil and spices.

Wash quinoa in saucepan then add boiled water. Add a few drops of olive oil. Bring to boil then simmer for 10 minutes. Cover completely and switch off heat. Leave on stove for another 10 minutes, then serve.

Serving suggestions: season with freshly ground pepper and salt. Add freshly cooked salmon or tin salmon if eating on the go. Place some chopped basil or herb of your choice topped with chopped BBQ chicken. Vegetarian-style will be added herb, chopped tomato, avocado, cucumber cubes, or grated carrot. Try steamed asparagus, kale, yellow squash mixed with chopped red onion, salt and pepper and a squeeze of olive oil, or just with a poached egg.

Winter Vegetable Soup

- 500g of gravy beef, cubed (optional)
- 3 carrots, cubed
- 2 turnips, chopped
- 2 parsnips, chopped
- 1 large brown onion, diced
- 4 to 5 stalks of celery, including tops, sliced
- ½ cup of red lentils (soak in boiled water and let stand for 30 minutes. Drain water and add more boiling water, and stand for another 30 minutes)
- ½ cup of green lentils (repeat above cooking process)

In a large heavy base pan, brown onion in a small amount of olive oil. Add beef cubes to onion and sprinkle with freshly ground pepper and cook for five minutes. Drain green and red lentils then add to pan. Cook for 15 minutes with lid on. Add some coarse sea salt and the rest of the vegetables. Add boiling water to cover all the vegetables and cook gently for two hours. Add water during cooking time. Serve and enjoy this hearty but light soup. When cooled pack the rest of the soup in small containers and store in the freezer for cooking-free nights.

Vegetable Stew

- 1 large brown onion, diced
- 1 to 2 tsp of curry powder
- 6 Brussel sprouts, halved
- 1 green capsicum, cut in small squares
- 125g of green beans, halved
- 1 or 2 zucchinis cut in thick slices, then cut each slice in 4 pieces
- ½ sweet potato, cubed
- Japanese or Kent pumpkin (1 to 2 cups full, thinly sliced)

Pour a small amount of olive oil in a large and deep frying pan or wok and gently brown onion. Add curry powder. Add small amount of water and the Japanese or Kent pumpkin. Cover and cook gently until reduced to a puree. Add the rest of the vegetables and simmer gently for 20 minutes. Serve with fresh salmon cutlets or lightly marinated chicken (see recipe below).

Marinated Chicken

- 500g chicken tenderloins or thickly sliced chicken breast (free range)
- Marinade:
- 2 tbsp Bragg All Purpose Seasoning from Soy Protein
- Freshly ground mixed pepper and sea salt
- A good sprinkle of olive oil
- Leaves from a few stems of thyme

Coat tenderloin or sliced chicken breast in marinade and let stand for 15 to 30 minutes (it won't matter if they are coated and cooked straight away, if pressed for time). Brown chicken in a frying pan with no added oil for 5 to 10 minutes on medium to high heat, turning pieces a few times. Then place lid on pan and turn stove off. Leave on hot plate for another 10 to 15 minutes before serving.

Garlic Sweet Potato and Green Beans

- 1 or 2 handfuls of green beans, halved
- 1 or 1/2 large yellow sweet potato, cubed
- 1 to 2 cloves of garlic crushed with salt
- ½ tsp each of caraway and cumin seeds, ground

In a large frying pan place butter, ghee, or olive oil. Add crushed garlic and sauté. Add sweet potato and green beans. Sprinkle with caraway and cumin, add salt then mix thoroughly. Add a small amount of boiled water and mix well. Cook gently for 15 to 20 minutes or until tender.

Eye Fillet Steak in Marinade

- 500g of eye fillet in one or two pieces
- 2 to 3 tbsp of Bragg All Purpose (BAPS), Seasoning from Soy Protein

- 1 clove of garlic, crushed with salt
- Freshly ground pepper
- 1 tbsp of olive oil

Marinate 1cm sliced steak in BAPS from soy protein with crushed garlic, olive oil, and pepper for 15 to 30 minutes.

Using high heat, brown meat on both sides. Place lid on frying pan. Turn stove off and allow meat to finish cooking in remaining heat. Stand for another 10 minutes before serving.

Green Lentils with Carrots

- ½ to 1 cup of green lentils (soaked in boiled water for 30 minutes, then repeat the process)
- 1 large red onion, diced or sliced
- 2 cloves of garlic + 1 small piece of ginger, crushed with a mortar and pestle
- 2 to 3 carrots, peeled and sliced
- A few sprigs of parsley

In a large saucepan, add a small amount of olive oil or ghee. Sauté crushed garlic, ginger and sliced onion. Add drained green lentils and carrots. Mix well. Add 1tsp Himalayan or sea salt and 2 cupsof boiling water. Mix well. Bring everything to the boil. Place lid halfway on saucepan and cook for one hour, stirring occasionally. Add water if necessary. Mix in fresh chopped parsley before serving.

Serve with brown rice or basmati rice, accompanied with a warm yellow squash salad or a tomato salsa with fresh coriander and chopped avocado.

Yellow Squash Salad

Steam 2 to 4 yellow squash, depending on the size. Cut in four or eight pieces. Add a good drop of olive oil and the juice of half a lemon or cider vinegar. Add some finely chopped red onion, some freshly grounded pepper and sea or Himalayan or sea salt and 2 cups of boiling water.

Tomato Salsa with Coriander

- 1 or 2 ripe tomatoes, diced finely
- 1 small brown or red onion (alternately 2 shallots), finely chopped
- A few sprigs of coriander, finely chopped

Mix well together. Season with freshly ground pepper and salt. Add to the mixture a squirt of olive oil, a few drops of sesame oil, and a dash of Tabasco sauce. Serve with rice dishes.

Leafy Greens and Rice

- Choko vine (upper part only). Cut soft stems in 3-4cm pieces as well as leaves
- 1 clove of garlic + 1 small piece of fresh or frozen ginger

Wash and drain stems and leaves. Add olive oil to hot pan. Crush ginger/garlic in a pestle and mortar with salt. Add ginger/garlic mixture and gently sauté without burning. Add ½ cup of boiling water to pan. Add cut up stems and leaves to pan. Bring to the boil. Season with sea or Himalayan salt. Mix well, then turn stove off. Leave on hot plate for 10 minutes, then serve with wild, basmati or brown rice, accompanied with a tomato salsa or even some choko or green mango or raw vegetable preserve. Addition to this dish can be a fried egg, parsley and onion omelette, or poached egg.

Chinese or English spinach, silverbeet, or beetroot tops can be cooked the same way. These dishes are healthy and cost nearly nothing to put together. It is really the simplest form of cooking. These are the types of foods I grew up on. It is definitely better than McDonald's. To prepare any salad, use your imagination and mix colours and textures to have a combination of taste. Add some walnuts, pine nuts or silvered almond for a crunchy effect and nutrition value. Avoid too much seasoning. Lemon or lime juice is always a good alternative to vinegar, unless it is cider vinegar. Add a dash of olive oil and it is all done.

Objection and responses:

I am not a good cook, preparing food is a chore.

Preparing food is easy. It is the buying and choosing what to eat that is a bigger process.

I am always busy and do not have time to cook or prepare food for myself.

Preparing food can take 15 to 30 minutes. Planning what to eat prior to purchasing will make this task a lot easier.

I rather someone else prepare my food for me.

That is fine. If you can have an agreement for someone to prepare or cook your meals in exchange for helping them with one of your skills, that should work perfectly. There are also a lot of companies who will supply weekly meals to you; 'Hello Fresh' will provide recipes and fresh ingredients. All you have to do is find someone to put it together for you.

3 actions to take as a result of reading this chapter:

1. See if someone close to you can provide fresh meals for you in exchange for other services. You can come to an agreement with someone and not miss out on nutritious meals.
2. Think fresh. The more you eat fresh, the more nutrition is available through what you eat and drink.
3. Eat simply, and mostly vegetarian, because it is best for the body and the mind. If you are of a Type a blood group you can eat meat occasionally. You will not miss out of protein since chia seed provides a high level of protein and other nutrients.

> 'I watch cooking change the cook, just as it transforms the food.'
> – Laura Esquivel

Nurture Yourself

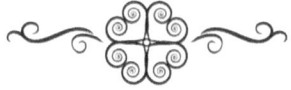

Love your body, love your life.

'We shall not cease from exploration and the end to all our exploring will be to arrive where we started and know the place for the first time.'

– T.S. Elliott

Keeping your body fit and healthy is the best gift you can give yourself. When we ensure that the body is operating to its optimum, we create joy and serenity in our life. It is great to practice putting yourself first, especially when life gets busy. Have a date with yourself and make sure that it is replenishing time for you; it could be time for planning, reading, walking on the beach, and even having a massage or a nice bath with essential oils and candles. As we spend some quality time with ourselves we get to recharge our battery so to function with efficiency, clarity, and purpose.

In contrast:
We may allow ourselves to be resigned and cynical about our life's situation. We can get caught up into work overload and other

commitments. We slide into the rut of being tired, stressed, overweight, and a life that is out of control. We can also allow ourselves to be beaten by the circumstances of life. The shocking truth is that you are the only person managing your life. What are you going to do about it?

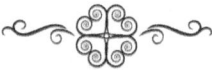

How important is it to plan and create a balanced lifestyle? Despite leading a busy life, and a demanding career or job, we need to have family time. When in a relationship it is very important to create time together, otherwise before long there may not be any relationship. Goalsetting and planning is what carves the structure to make everything happen the way it is scheduled. It is also about commitment and what takes precedence in someone's life. Anything is possible as long as it is created. This is all about sealing our intention so it can be manifested.

Nurturing ourselves is a must to avoid being sick and burning out, and therefore avoiding being looked after by other people. It allows us to give the best of ourselves and to others. This includes keeping up with good nutrition and an exercise regime to keep the body healthy. Minimise the routine of buying already-cooked meals. Practice a nutritious and balanced diet routine, or get a health coach. It may sometimes be quicker to go home and prepare a wholesome salad instead of waiting in a queue for some bought unhealthy meals.

Nurturing is not only about balancing the mind and body, but also by keeping tabs on your emotions. How do we do that when things get a bit chaotic? The first thing to do is take a deep breath. The second thing to do is to accept what is happening. We sometimes do not have control over certain circumstances in our life. In these frustrating times, it is best to not react to what is happening. One way to do that is by disengaging and walking away, thus allowing time to find a solution. If the solution is not found, it may be time to reach out and talk about it with someone or put it down on paper.

Nurturing yourself can also mean going away on a trip to change your environment and come back to see everything with fresh eyes. It means spending some time away from home or doing something that is not part of a very rigid routine. It means visiting friends and going to a get together, or attending a party to chill out. It is about going to a concert, the movies, or listening to some soothing and relaxing music. It can also mean going on a dinner date in a first-class restaurant.

It is also nice to create a community that gets to support you in time of need, a group to connect with when not attending to business or dealing with earning a dollar. It means that you shift into a more relaxed mode and turn your attention towards those who enjoy your company. It becomes a time to laugh and have light conversations. It is a time of connection and contribution, discovering something new in each other and celebrating it.

Another way of nurturing yourself is to practice yoga and meditation regularly. The word yoga means 'to harness'. By practicing yoga, we facilitate the movement of 'prana' and 'apana', which are positive and negative energy, through the nerve channels (nadis). This process unblocks and purifies the nerve channels keeping the vital energy circulating throughout the body. It provides the link between the astral and physical body. The nerve channels (nadis) are all connected to the sympathetic and parasympathetic division of the autonomic nervous system.

Observing the chakras helps make the connection between our physical and spiritual being, because we are vibration and energy we can achieve optimum health and vitality at any time. We are responsible for maintaining our energy bank to activate our healing whenever our body needs it.

The Seven Chakras

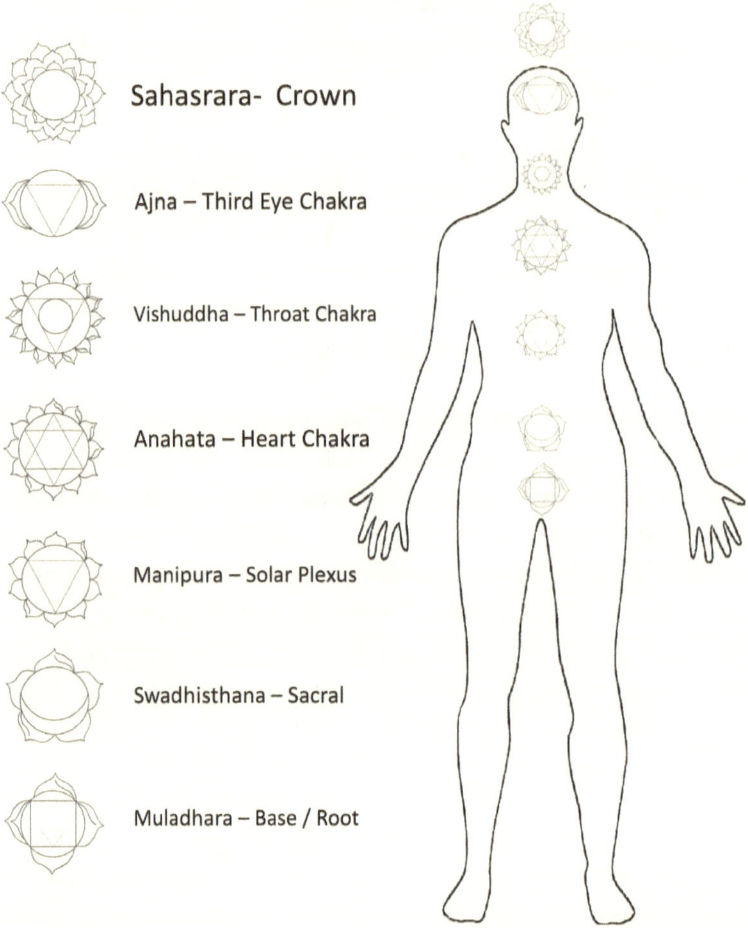

Sahasrara – Crown

Ajna – Third Eye Chakra

Vishuddha – Throat Chakra

Anahata – Heart Chakra

Manipura – Solar Plexus

Swadhisthana – Sacral

Muladhara – Base / Root

 'OM' – the eternal word from Sanskrit meaning: 'What was, what is and what shall be'. This powerful symbol represents the dream state, the waking state, the deep dreamless sleep, topped with 'Maya – the veil of illusion' and the dot representing the transcendental state.

The Path to Enlightenment
The Seven Chakras – Centres of Energy in the Astral body

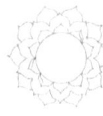 Sahasrara- Crown Chakra

Thousand-petalled Chakra
When kundalini reaches this point through yoga practices and meditation, one attains samādi (super consciousness)

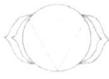 Ajna – Third Eye Chakra

Two-petalled Chakra
Seat of the Mind
– Mantra is OM

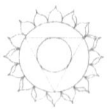 Vishuddha – Throat Chakra

Sixteen petalled Chakra
Element is Ether
– Mantra is Ham

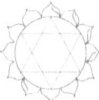 Anahata – Heart Chakra

Twelve petalled Chakra
Element is Air
– Mantra is Yam

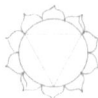 Manipura – Solar Plexus

Ten petalled Chakra
Element is Fire
– Mantra is Ram

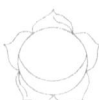 Swadhisthana – Sacral

Six petalled Chakra
Element is Water
– Mantra is Vam

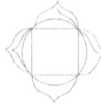 Muladhara – Base / Root
Where the 'Ida' and 'Pingala nadis' are located allowing 'Kundalini' (static cosmic energy) to flow through the chakras alongside the 'Sushumna' the spinal cord.

Four petalled Chakra
Element is Earth
– Mantra is Lam

The Seven Chakras

Linked with the sympathetic and parasympathetic divisions of the body through the spinal cord.

Chakra	Associated With
Sahasrara – Crown	Super consciousness
Ajna – Third Eye Chakra	Brain / Pineal / Pituitary
Vishuddha – Throat Chakra	Thyroid / Parathyroid
Anahata – Heart Chakra	Thymus / Heart / Lung
Manipura – Solar Plexus	Pancreas / Spleen / Kidney / Adrenals
Swadhisthana – Sacral	Sexual Organs (Gonads)
Muladhara – Base / Root	Base of Spine – Sacrum

The Tree of Life - Connection to 7 Chakras

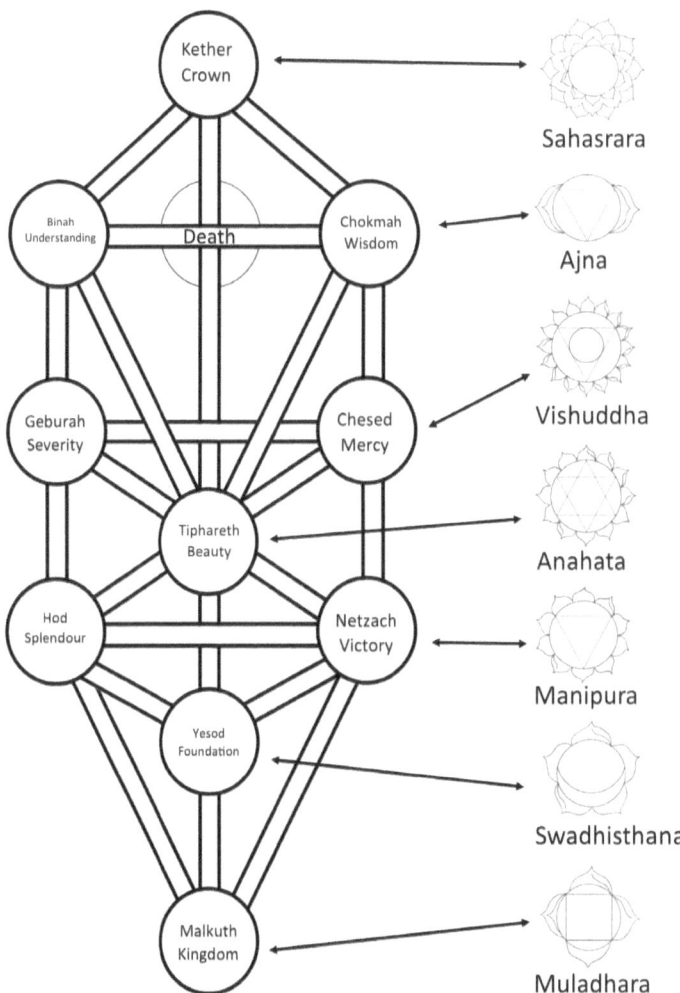

Objections and responses:

What if I work long hours and do not get to have time for myself?

It is so important to find time, whether it is taking a short walk at lunchtime, listening to some soft music in the car, or having a herbal tea or a glass of wine before cooking dinner. It is imperative to create that time for yourself.

What if I have to take care of my family? I would hate to neglect them.

That is fine. Include everyone in what needs to done so you are not the only one doing all the tasks. Delegate while you have a 15 minute break for a meditation or an aromatic bath.

I do not like asking for help, I'd rather do things myself.

Letting go of control is liberating. It creates trust and allows others to contribute to you. It is about acceptance and sharing. It is about loving and being loved.

3 actions to take as a result of reading this chapter:

1. Schedule set times to work and play.
2. Nurturing time is a must, whether it is 15 minutes, 30 minutes, one hour or one day.
3. Monitor what you give out, creating a balance that will see you manage yourself and others with ease and grace.

> 'You are that which you have been seeking. Just relax and sit around the warmth of your own heart.'
> – Brandon Bays

Your Quest

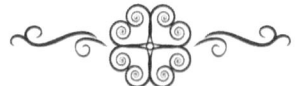

Your assignment is to discover who you really are.

> 'Knowing yourself is the beginning of all wisdom.'
> – Aristotle

Who am I as a human being? It's not always easy to get an answer. Some have found the answer but some are still searching. This is your main assignment while on Earth. It can take a lifetime to discover who we really are and what our purpose on this planet. Some already know whilst in their mother's womb. Yet many leave this planet not having figured out who they were or what was their purpose on this planet.

Yes, life is a mystery. Coming from a large family, it took me a while to figure out why I am here, but now I get it. But I have to say that it has not been easy for me. For years I had not been present to what is here within me. I have been side-tracked and pursuing things outside of me, hoping I will get there. Every single moment of our lives we have clues coming to us, not all of us listen. So look, listen, and learn. We learn every day from people who enter our life.

Everyone we meet acts as a mirror image of who we are. These are the people who become our teachers. When this occur we have to learn not to react but to take note on what is being shown to us. It may be something that we are being called to look at so we can transform our life. So, don't shoot the messenger. It is best to thank them for the learning and move on. I always say that every bit of information that comes to us, whether good or bad, is good information. It helps us learn what we like and what we do not like about ourselves.

In contrast:
We may hold on to an incident that has happened. We create our own version of it and that becomes our own story. We may talk or think about it a lot. It can consume our life to the point that we are willing to give it all our energy and miss out on living a life that rocks. This gets stored in our memory cells and we react each time something or someone reminds us of it (usually around the full moon). We end up being its victim, totally unaware of the little prison we have built for ourselves.

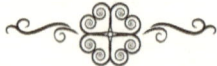

The Macrobiotics Principles is based on Oriental medicine dating back more than 5000 years. Zen Macrobiotic is a guide to rediscover the ancient basic truths about optimum health and longevity. It teaches the human species how to find happiness through having a healthy lifestyle and achieving youthfulness through nutrition. Macrobiotics is the basis of the biological application of Oriental philosophy and medicine. It is about taking responsibility for not only yourself but also for your environment so everything and everyone coexists in a harmonious way. It is about gratitude and appreciation for this amazing planet that provides us with everything we could wish for. It is about discovering authentic happiness.

As we go back to the teachings of the Far East we discover the philosophy on how to bring back balance and equilibrium to the planet. For decades we trusted professionals, like doctors, teachers, and even nuns and priests to advise and guide us on our way. Some of these professionals have themselves faltered or lost their way. The world is not prospering but instead falling into more chaos and uncertainty. Hospitals are getting larger and we are training more nurses and doctors to look after more sick people. We are building more mental health facilities, prisons, and recruiting more police to keep law and order. We are far from being free as a society, nor do we feel that there is any justice in the world. The education system may not be enough to teach us the things we need as human beings. We can become too attached to money, fame, and success but all these things do not necessarily bring us happiness.

I have known about the yin-yang principles for a long time, and have applied it throughout my life. I have not been too rigid with it, but is has been a good guide especially when I was diagnosed with Type II diabetes. This philosophy helps us get more control or better management in balancing the acid and alkaline level in our body. Depending on our body type we can be more yin than yang. Whether we are male or female we can still have an imbalance of yin and yang in the body. As a rule, females are yin whereas males are yang. Everything we intake as nourishment can change our body chemistry at any time. Each fruit or vegetable can either be alkaline or acid. Tomatoes and potatoes, for example, are very yin (acid) so I totally avoid these two vegetables, especially since being prone to diabetes. When the body is too acidic we start to get sick.

It takes a constant effort to balance our diet on a daily basis but once we are in a routine the body easily adapts, then we start to enjoy the food that we know will contribute to our health. This is the reason why I started to follow the blood type diet a few years ago. It helps me balance my weight, keep away from foods that are not healthy for me, and I thoroughly enjoy the food that I choose to eat.

Another concept is the Ayurvedic medicine. Ayurveda comes from Sanskrit, meaning 'Science of Life'. It originates from India more than 5000 years ago, prior to the pyramids being built in Egypt. Ayurveda offers control over health and mind, ensuring a state of wellbeing and the capacity to extend the lifespan. It educates in restoring health when struck by sickness. It teaches how to balance the body, and to improve our immunity against viruses and diseases. By following these principles we can avoid heart attacks and keep our blood sugar and cholesterol at a normal level.

There is no need to survive on a handful of tablets at each meal to keep us alive in the 7th or 8th decade of our life. It is not necessary to follow rigorous diets or extreme exercise to keep healthy. Most people take daily vitamins that are not even suited for their health at times. Our body is designed to use its own pharmacy. Vitamins and supplements can be used to kick the body back into gear again but it has to be correctly prescribed, it pays to do research and seek advice. By taking the wrong vitamins we may be creating an imbalance in the body. Arthritis, diabetes, fibromyalgia, and other chronic inflammations diseases can be avoided by implementing only a few changes in the daily routine. Cancer can potentially be cured instead of being classified as a terminal illness.

These ancient philosophies have been guiding me along the way to find some answers about life. Having optimum health on a spiritual, mental, and physical level is imperative to make the best of our life on this planet. Things happen to us at times that we do not anticipate. These are the challenges that come our way to test our skills, and as we pass the tests we go to the next level. For us to learn our biggest lessons in life it is best not to react but to take on the learning instead. It is all about controlling our emotions. It takes some time to acquire wisdom. This comes with many lessons. Life is all about trial and error. It is about being ready to learn without judgement. It is about being thankful for every little thing in life. It is also about accepting things the way they are; knowing that everything is perfect in their imperfection.

Before we can heal the planet, we have to heal ourselves. Unless we have a vision about what we want for ourselves in life, we are unlikely to succeed. We must learn to look out for others. We live in a world of excessive waste and high pollution, and that needs to be corrected. We are all responsible for this planet. We cannot let it perish or we will perish with it.

Objections and responses:

Wouldn't it be simpler if we knew at the beginning what life is all about?
We are unique individuals. We all have to discover something special about ourselves.

Some geniuses have been able to work out what life is all about. Why can't we all do that?
We are given a life to make of it what we wish. We are capable to create the life that is right for us.

Life is tough sometimes. Why is that?
Part of you is a Super Being. Included in your assignment is to discover the Super Being within you. Then you will get the necessary clue on how to turn your obstacles into triumphs.

3 actions to take as a result of reading this chapter:
1. Keep searching for what you want for yourself until you find it. If you are determined enough it will come to you.
2. Instead of searching on the outside for what makes you happy, connect with you inner being find the answers that will be given to you.
3. Pay attention to the magic of the people around. They are your mirrors and act as your messengers. Do not react to them. Learn from them.

> 'I choose to make the rest of my life the best of my life.' – Louise Hay

Ten Rules For Being Human

Rule One: You will receive a body.
You may love it or hate it, but it will be yours for the duration of your life on Earth.

Rule Two: You will be presented with lessons.
You are enrolled in a full-time informal school called 'life.' Each day in this school you will have the opportunity to learn lessons. You may like the lessons or hate them, but you have designed them as part of your curriculum.

Rule Three: There are no mistakes, only lessons.
Growth is a process of experimentation, a series of trials, errors, and occasional victories. The failed experiments are as much a part of the process as the experiments that work.

Rule Four: A lesson is repeated until learned.
Lessons will be repeated to you in various forms until you have learned them. When you have learned them, you can then go on to the next lesson.

Rule Five: Learning does not end.
There is no part of life that does not contain lessons. If you are alive, there are lessons to be learned.

Rule Six: 'There' is no better than 'here'.
When your 'there' has become a 'here,' you will simply obtain a 'there' that will look better to you than your present 'here'.

Rule Seven: Others are only mirrors of you.
You cannot love or hate something about another person unless it reflects something you love or hate about yourself.

Rule Eight: What you make of your life is up to you.
You have all the tools and resources you need. What you do with them is up to you.

Rule Nine: Your answers lie inside of you.
All you need to do is look, listen, and trust.

Rule Ten: You will forget all of this at birth.
You can remember it if you want by unravelling the double helix of inner knowing.

Author and Coach Cherie Carter-Scott, from If Life is a Game, These are the Rules.

Time Indulgence

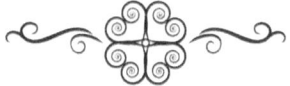

How would you like to find 10 hours to indulge in each and every week?

'The bad news is time flies. The good news is you're the pilot.'
– Michael Altshuler

How can we create more time to be with our family when it seems that we are fitting more and more in our week? Planning is one of the most important thing to donate your time to for you end up creating more time for yourself. The end result is that less time gets wasted and more tasks get achieved.

Team building or delegating is another time saver. So many small business owners I meet are reluctant to explore delegating tasks to others because they don't trust anyone else completing things their way. I find that this holds them back so much that they are unable to progress, evolve, or expand their business as much as they deserve to. Perfectionists want to do things in a specific way, thus creating more work for themselves and less time for them to indulge in things they love to do. I have been one for so many years and realise that it created more pain than joy in my life.

When letting others participate in things that we do, it enables us to allocate more time to things that needs our attention and skills. We can step up in the bigger roles and dedicate our time to what we are meant to do. It eventually give us the freedom to be with the people we love spending time with.

The best way to save on time is to create strategies to get more done in the shortest amount of time. Setting goals is a very efficient way for training the brain to get to tasks faster and economise on time. If we do not give our brains the right instructions it will pick up on any distractions to keep us busy; we end up creating things that we don't want. Once you have locked in your brain what needs to be done, it will get to the task and make it happen.

According to statistics, multitasking takes four times longer for you to complete any task compared to putting your time and effort on one task at a time. Very few people are able to multitask and achieve positive results. These people will either have machines or software programmes to help them in their tasks.

In contrast:
Having to deal with too many things at one time creates a lack of focus. One can be caught up in a state of chaos where nothing works. Valuing your time means avoiding long tasks that eats into your precious time. In some situations you end up going backwards and having to start all over again, which is such a waste of time.

When we are committed to achieve a task we give our word to, we ensure that we get to honour our word. Whether we are working for someone or working in our own business, honouring one's word means having integrity with oneself. This prevents us from getting into a state of procrastination, ensuring instead that we stay on purpose and complete things on time.

By focusing on specific tasks you get to reach your target in the shortest period of time. As time goes on we tend to do things differently. The systems that have been used in the past may not always be the best ways to save on time. As we merge more into the world of technology things are moving faster and it is becoming a challenge to keep up with things. Unfortunately for those who are not up-to-date with technology it can become a time-consuming exercise or even an impossible task. As a result we are being forced to redefine the way we do business. We have new entrepreneurs emerging with new business ideas all the time. Time allocation keeps changing to accommodate new roles as they are being created.

The marketing world is also changing, giving priority to digital media. Whether we are an organisation or a small business, networking is also becoming prominent and a way to move forward in the arena of business. Social media such as Facebook, Pinterest, and Instagram are being used widely in businesses. It saves time and money, resulting in a more efficient way of targeting a wider audience or market. This also allows one to reach out to the international market.

Competition has given way to collaboration. We can now find the experts who will train us in the skills we are seeking and exchange services. The world is shifting at such a fast pace that it gets to be exciting, overwhelming and opening up to endless opportunities

Time is what we use, to keep track on our planet. The human brain can only remember so much in a short time. It is said that our brain processes 400 billion bits of information every second, yet we are aware of only 2000 of them at any time. This is the main reason why we write goals, carry a diary, and have a planner. This ensures that whatever happens or whatever distraction we have does not pull us away from the life of our dreams.

When we look at ourselves as eternal beings we go beyond time. In that world, time does not exist. What creates our experience of time is the phenomenon of Earth spinning on its axis around the sun. It is also referred to as 'space-time continuum'.

People who have a few deadlines to meet would say, 'I am running out of time', forgetting the law of nature – what we say or think, we create. These people are constantly trying to beat time. As a result of their own interpretation of time it seems that the clock moves faster for them. Their biological reaction to time creates a physical response and create a heartrate that beats faster, their blood pressure would rise accordingly, and their sugar level would also be affected.

Whereas people who live like they have all the time in the world end up with less stress and living longer. Our perception of time depends on how we manage it. By restructuring our perception of time we can restructure the physical expression of the body. We are able then, to delay or even reverse the aging process.

Our sensory experience of time is always determined on what is happening with each of us on a mental, physical, and emotional level. It all goes back to thoughts. Have you ever sat somewhere and got lost in your thoughts, realising that two hours have passed by you and you had even forgotten where you were? We can determine what time means to us according to how we want to live and what we want to create, or achieve. People who are money-driven create $10 million in one sentence through an idea and it is done. Any amount of money can be created through hard work or smart work. Ideally, strategy and planning are the best ways to create time and use it constructively.

I personally have not used a watch for at least 10 years. I do everything using my senses and am guided by the Universe. I also can tell the time fairly accurately by glancing at the clock a few times and sticking to how I have planned my day. I find if I set my intention prior to my appointments I usually remain punctual. I always set my alarm to wake up on time for the earlier engagement of the day. I find that by just creating the intention before I sleep, I get to wake up five or 10 minutes before my alarm goes off. In other words, I create my own time.

I have known a time where every minute counted. I worked in the corporate world where punctuality, impeccability, and efficiency were paramount. I was able to keep on track and dance in the chaos of that world. In those days, I practically felt indestructible. This is the reason why I convinced myself that I was going to get my marriage right and it would all be ok in the end. Little did I realise at the time that staying in a destructive relationship and putting up with domestic violence for 20 years was totally insane. It shows that the way my brain was wired then was not the way I see things today. I no longer carry these beliefs.

Years later, I told myself that I wasted my time and so many years of my life. But I also got to learn that we cannot reverse time. These were life lessons and no matter how painful my experience was I had to go through it all to be where I am now. It was all part of the contract. Fortunately, I managed to have other strategies that allowed me to cope with that situation and survive it all. I can see now how attending yoga classes and spending time studying helped me escape the madness in my life and kept me in touch with real time.

During those years I was working full-time, studying part-time. I was travelling many kilometres daily by public transport. Life was insane but everything always fell into place somehow. As my son was growing up I used to fit so much in each day. I created time to go to and from the babysitters, then to morning and afternoon school care, then to football practices, games or other sporting activities. When we need time, we make it all happen.

Concerning time we have to create a shift in our consciousness. At all times we must be aware that time is relevant to what phase of life we are going through. We have to constantly reassess time to match our goals and the results we want to get. As you put your goals in place, you must set a time limit to when you want to achieve it, visualise what it would look like then and how you would have transformed to enjoy it.

As the world transforms, we learn to transform with it. Although we know that most of the time we are drawn to the past instead of living in the present moment, being present is where we must be at all times as this is where all the living and the learning takes place. This is the time that matters the most.

Getting back to the real world, the world of form, where we have to take action to make things happen, what is required from us is being in control. To get the desired result in our life and minimise suffering we have to set our intentions.

Primarily we must convert our intentions into goals which are written with precise and clear instructions accompanied with visualisation and the right emotions for when they come into life. Reading your goals every day will keep you focused on achieving them faster. Writing in your journal will also keep you on track. When you are playing a big game you can start planning or filling your diary for the next 6-12 months. Some people will even start recording the following year's goals and listen to it every day.

As a routine I tend to deal with the next day by planning it the night before and have it fresh in my mind what type of outcome I am creating for myself, especially when dealing with challenging situations. Some weeks may be full of appointments or commitments. It is fruitful to mentally go through your week ahead on the Sunday night to see what needs to be addressed. It helps to juggle things easily if anything unforeseen crops up. It helps eliminate stress and ensures productivity, thus helps you keep on top of things.

Does time really exist? Time is a relative phenomenon. Nothing is ever created in the past or the future; it is always in the present moment. Everything happens in the now – the eternal moment. It is said that in the gap between each of our experiences in the material world is what we perceive time to be. Nevertheless, however we experience time, whether we perceive time as going too fast or too slow, in reality time is infinite.

Objections and responses:

I have set goals and they do not work for me.
Have you written your goals in the present moment and do you believe that they are achievable?

I do not like a planner. It is too much work and I do not have time for it.
Without a planner or anything concrete to keep you on track you will be caught in the vortex called life and you might not achieve as much as you would like to.

I start putting things in place and then it becomes too hard to keep a routine.
We all experience this. This is part of being human. Do not let this deter you. If you want to play a big game you will have to be instrumental in creating something that will produce the best results. They say there is no gain without pain. In a way this is true because without effort there isn't any good results.

3 actions to take as a result of reading this chapter:
1. Get a diary for the next year as soon as it is available in the shops and start planning all the things you dream of and would like to have in your life.
2. Do a vision board with bold and colourful pictures, making it daring and beyond your imagination. Apart from your monthly goals write your one year, three year, and five year goals.
3. Regularly check on where you are at with them. Review what you have to put in place to get closer to them and celebrate the ones you have achieved.

> 'All we have to do is decide what to do with the time that is given to us.'
> – J.R.R Tolkien

Total Transformation

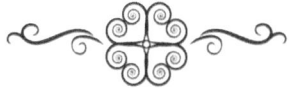

When we react to what happens around us we create suffering.

'Whatever suffering arises has a reaction as its cause. If all reactions cease to be then there is no more suffering.'
– Buddha

Looking at the following five points we can consider what transformation means:

- How can we have a better understanding on how to reduce our suffering and create mental balance and calm in our life.
- Instead of trying to avoid pain we learn to observe as it arises and passes away.
- We can learn about Vipassana and the law of impermanence.
- As the world outside is constantly changing, so does everything inside our mind and body.
- As one transforms oneself, one transform the world. This is our main responsibility.

In contrast:
Not considering that we have a role to play on this planet. We carry on with our own selfish ways and expect the world to contribute to us instead in contributing to it. We do not take on our responsibility in managing our mental, physical, emotional and spiritual wellbeing.

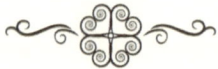

What we discover with Vipassana meditation is that it liberates us from conditions of the past. As we become aware of these conditions we learn to release them instead of carrying them around in our DNA. Otherwise we get triggered whenever they come to the surface. We can easily learn methods of releasing what is no longer serving us and replace it with the right energy that will contribute to our growth.

As we learn to be responsible for the type of energy we carry with us we can change the energy in our environment. As we work towards the path to enlightenment we get to fulfil our contribution to humanity and to the world. We get to end the game of avoiding the unpleasant sensations or feelings and constantly seeking the pleasant ones. We give up the never ending rounds of push and pull, including the misery that comes with attraction and repulsion.

When we enter this world, our first ever experience is crying. If we fail to cry at the time, to make sure we are breathing and alive we get our first smack on the bottom to have us experience our first breath. Because we have not yet discovered the world of language then, the only form of communication as a baby is crying. When babies need feeding, burping, or a nappy change, crying is the only form of asking. Then comes the suffering from colic, constipation, teething, and so on.

As a toddler there are new experiences likes falls, injuries, and not having things our way. As we move on through the stages of childhood to adolescence and adulthood, there are more disappointments and lots more tears. Although generally males and females deal with their emotions in totally different ways, but as human beings we are all affected by the challenges of life. Whether it is tears of joy or sorrow, it becomes very part of life. Our life oscillates constantly between pain and pleasure.

Human suffering and unhappiness, as the Buddha teaches us, mainly come from attachment and craving. As we grow up we get addicted to craving and desire. We can get stuck into a world of always wanting to get somewhere, seeking a world of perfection or attaining something. We live in an endless world of wanting more. In the end it seems that we can never get there. We crave fast food and fast cars, or lots of alcohol and plenty of coffee to dull the pain of not being able to get what we want on a daily basis. We live in a world of looking good and always wanting the best. There is a price to pay for everything and the cost could sometimes be too high. I've heard someone say, 'You can have whatever you want, but be willing to pay the price'. In the long run, cravings become habit and then turn into addiction.

Life is an experience and the idea is to tap into our best qualities to survive the most painful parts of it. When Jesus came to earth, His message was, 'Love one another' yet through religion we can make ourselves wrong. We tend to live in the world of 'good' and 'bad' because that is what we were taught. We end up in a state of guilt and shame that does not give us anything to recreate ourselves with. With all this comes isolation and the fear of being judged. Most of those who have big challenges feel alone and unsupported, some end up committing suicide. When being stuck in the victim mode, we rob ourselves of years of enrichment, love, sharing, and happiness.

As we look for answers we eventually realise that there is more to life than the negative side. We learn to reach out and ask for help and when we do, help is always on its way – 'When the student is ready, the teacher appears'. Motivational speakers talk a lot about the 'Law of Attraction'. When we shift our mindset we turn our attention to who we really are and the role we are meant to play. We discover that life on this planet is not about us, but about the people around us. For that to take place we must primarily deal with the past and let bygone be bygone. This action of letting go can be difficult and quite painful. It is a big transition. Shifting from a victim mode to finding love and abundance through forgiveness is transforming and liberating.

I have seen many people who are angels, mentors, adoring parents, dedicated family members, and friends who guide others smoothly through life's challenges. These are the amazing human beings who are compassionate and generous and ready to assist those who have not had a rosy life. Whether we like it or not, the reality is that we live in a world of suffering. In the past I was always experiencing confusion, and trying to find the logic behind things that happened to me.

I relied on my faith to comfort me, telling myself that if I made enough sacrifices then there was bound to be a reward. I realised that with religion and traditions came judgement. As I got older I gradually found answers to so many questions I had been asking myself.

I understood that my struggle with my marriage was also influenced by my religious beliefs. Like many others, I imagine, I stayed in a destructive marriage for too long. My marital situation also had me questioning my faith for a long time. Who was God really? Why does he allow such unfairness in life? Why do many people get away with what they do?

Whilst dealing with the domestic violence I had to tap into my inner knowing and the strength within to pull me out of such misery. As I kept asking God and the Universe for help, I was led to an amazing woman who became my therapist and mentor who taught me so much. My spiritual journey had just begun and I have not stopped learning since then. I had finally unlocked and started using my toolbox to discover many facets of happiness, joy and contentment.

In her book *Sacred Contracts* Caroline Myss explains how we all have a sacred contract to fulfil when we come to Earth. From my understanding it is a contract with God, our Creator or the Divine, The Master of the Universe. In her book she also describes the sacred contracts between God and the four major Spiritual Masters; Abraham, Jesus – Son of God and Son of Man, Muhammed, and Buddha. These spiritual masters still impact humanity today with their teachings. All of them shared an awakening process. They were mentored, then underwent tests that challenged their soul over the strength of their ego.

When we look at the law of impermanence and the teachings of Buddha, we realise that we can have some control over the suffering in our life. Everything that our five senses detects gets processed mentally, which creates a physical reaction in our body and causing a sensation. Each of these reactions get created via the electromagnetic and biochemical process in our body that happens moment by moment. This is the way mind and matter manifests itself. It is not permanent and is always changing.

Just as the world outside is constantly changing so does everything inside ourselves, mentally and physically. Any effort to hold on to something that is constantly changing gets to be beyond our control and results in suffering. When we get to see that this world is transitionary and that attachment to anything is fruitless, then we get to consider letting go of the suffering. This is also true about any physical pain. The more we focus on the pain, the more intense it becomes. When we step back and become the observer of the pain, it dissipates.

We live in an ignorant world of like and dislikes – a world of judgement. This way of being creates a chain of events. How can we break this chain of cause and effect? As we surrender to this world of craving and aversion we mechanically get attached to it as it multiplies and intensifies, causing more misery in the future. All this eventually converts to strong emotions that end up overpowering our conscious mind. At that point our best judgement is swept aside, giving way to unpleasant words and actions. Such blind reactions at that moment brings much suffering and misery to ourselves and people we really love.

By breaking the barrier between the conscious and the unconscious mind we are able to observe the sensation in the body. Meditation makes us conscious of our body awareness and sensations. Meditation allow our quiet mind to connect with our inner being and away from the ego. We get to observe the pain without reaction. Since the body is made of vibrations, the pain arises and passes away. The body then becomes more supple and flexible and the mind more balanced resulting in you becoming master of your own self and the pain cannot master you.

Concerning the world of mind and matter, it is said that the body is made of atoms and matter. It seems as being nothing but subtle wavelets of subatomic particles. Whenever a thought enters our mind, it is accompanied with a physical sensation. As the solidity of mind and body dissolves, what remains is the oscillation and vibration from what we experience as the mental formation of mind and matter. Because it rapidly arises and passes away, what we may experience is flow of vibration or a current moving through our physical body.

Out of countless beings in the Universe it seems that we are more focused on the 'I' – the self. As we seek fulfilment and happiness we merge our wants and fears to imprison ourselves from the rest of the world. By emerging from this self-obsession we release ourselves from our illusion and become aware of the ephemeral nature of the world and the 'self'.

As we increase our awareness, it allows us to contribute to a transforming world. Living in the world as an observer and not reacting to what goes on outside ourselves, we can spend more time changing what is inside ourselves. Our responsibility lies in what we bring into the world as it creates a ripple effect. As we learn to be compassionate but not attached to people and events in the world we can be instrumental in nurturing love, peace, and harmony.

Objections and responses:

I do not have time for meditation.

Meditation can take as little at 15 minutes or as long as two hours, or longer. You may choose to do what works for you.

I have my own religion and do not believe in meditation or yoga.

Meditation does not interfere with any religion; even prayer is considered a form of meditation. Yoga is a form of exercise that is not only beneficial to the outer part of the body but also to the internal organs, keeping them healthy.

I do not believe that people should get away with what they do wrong.

People can lead their life the way they choose to and it is not for us to pass judgement. We can choose to detach from them and from what they do.

3 actions to take as a result of reading this chapter:
1. Take time to meditate regularly, it will have you discover clarity in making decisions and having access to freedom and peace of mind.
2. When someone has said or done something to you, pull away and take time to observe your reaction as you deal with it, then let it go.
3. Self-development plays a big part in learning. As people share their own experiences we can accept our own vulnerability.

> 'We must always change, renew, rejuvenate ourselves; otherwise we harden.'
> – Goethe

Global Shift

Creating 1000 years of peace on Earth

'Think globally rather than locally. People who look different, who speak a different language, who have different beliefs – are a part of US. We are all in now-here together.'
– Wayne Dyer

The world is constantly changing and evolving. We are starting to let go of some traditional ways and moving to a more unified way of connecting and accepting others.

The spiritual awakening of the planet sees many structures being dismantled. The business world is constantly reinventing itself as we advance in this new century. Someone once said, 'We do not need more money, but we need better ideas'. Facebook, one of the most successful media companies, does not even have to create content for its clients. Uber provides transport to its customers and does not have to pay any cost in vehicle maintenance. Airbnb does not own any real estate and yet successfully provides accommodation to many happy customers around the world.

For those who have known scarcity, now they are discovering abundance. The world of collaboration is opening the doors to generous entrepreneurs reaching out to many. They are creating ways of doing business with win/win situations.

In contrast:
We can bury our heads in the sand and keep conforming to old ways that do not work. When resisting change and wanting to control, we create more suffering and the world does not progress. Instead of going forward, we go backward and create misery.

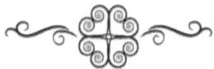

The global shift is happening because it is inevitable. As we understand that we do not have to be driven by fear any longer we can live a life of purpose and passion, starting with practicing a non-judgemental approach to anything and anyone. As a collective we observe and adopt more tolerance and compassion in our world which ends up creating a ripple effect.

Once upon a time it was everyone for oneself, but there has been a shift in the human consciousness. We have to realise that this battle is not to be fought as individuals, but as a world community. Social media allows so much freedom in self-expression within communities around the world. Facebook has strict guidelines that allows this form of social media to be a way of reaching out and being of service to the community. As a result it is seeing people being supported as they need it. Businesspeople are becoming smart entrepreneurs willing to collaborate with each other and creating a more harmonious way of serving each other and the community. This platform was created to bring communities together, dismissing force, elevating individual power, and exploring limitlessness.

We tend to be attached to our views and beliefs. We are convinced that our views are the only ones that count. It seems to be the same with traditions. As we grow up, traditions keeps us in a way of life that we feel cannot change. There comes a point when tradition gives way to evolution.

We had been relying on churches, therapists, the police, or the government as authorities to guide and help us. We are seeing dramatic changes allowing the individual more freedom and self-expression. The power of self-expression is now liberating human beings from their prison of mind and body. As the sharing happens, the healing is being done instantly. The non-profit organisations are taking over roles that the government have failed in. They are playing a huge role in the community and filling in the gap where government do not provide the necessary help.

As we are connected to a whole Universe, we are being provided with everything we need to have a successful life in this world. We have our own toolbox to make this journey the most amazing experience. We are now tapping into all this knowledge that has always existed within ourselves. The power of communication opens new avenues. Instead of relying on people in authority to give us the right information to move forward we discover that most of it is readily accessible through other avenues. For decades we had to either buy information or services to improve or remedy any situations we were dealing with. Today, practically any information we need is readily available on Google. We are equipped with the intelligence that is more powerful that we can imagine. It has always been there but we have been blinded and made to believe for years that we did not have it or it did not exist.

Many teachers and healers have been instrumental in bringing much healing to the planet after the devastating wars and destruction in the world. The human race has gone through so much suffering. Many spiritual teachers have come along and taken part in healing the world. I spent many years on self-development and self-healing. We have recently lost two famous motivational and dedicated human beings, Wayne Dyer and Louise Hay. They played a huge part in changing mindsets and helping people rediscover their own healing powers. We can now start to heal and show others to do the same. The motivational speakers who are still with us like Tony Robbins, Bob Proctor, and Caroline Myss are still helping transform the planet today.

As we get awakened we have many spiritual healers and teachers who are passionate about healing the planet. As we get awakened there are more teachers arising to serve humanity. It seems the human psyche is ready to embrace a shift in consciousness and heal the human beings on this planet. We are geared towards the same goal guided by the new generations that are already embracing it fully. As there is more humility in the world from those who have lost much of what they once owned, the world is shifting to a better place. Many have given up their corporate career, successful status, and their wealth to just follow their passion of being in sync with humanity and its everyday needs. We are well on our way to save the world!

The main teaching in self-development today is about being wealthy. This is manifesting itself everywhere, but the real wealth, it seems, is about shifting the money and distributing it where it is needed the most. There does not seem to be categories of who should have the money or not. Those who have had the millions are losing it and those who have never experienced it are now having a taste of it. Fortunately, those who keep attaining their financial goals are wisely giving their time and money to allow many others to take part in this revolutionary world of wealth and success.

The healers of the world in the roles of coaches and natural health therapists have been sent to us to assist us in healing the past. When we heal ourselves we're supporting those who are hurting, providing them with an access to reach out for the help they need for their healing. People who have suffered abuse, rape, and other atrocities are breaking their silence and calling out those offenders, keeping them accountable. These brave humans are speaking out and telling their stories, and are free again.

It is no longer shameful to ask for assistance. Today it seems that asking for help is a natural way of being with a community to get the support needed instead of having to fight to survive. There is justice finally happening in the world and the victims are now becoming the victors. Those who do not see the opportunity in implementing change are not ready for growth. Being available to assist without judgement is paramount; it creates access to those who are readily open for help. Fear can be a great factor for some people who are not ready to open up. As we tend to stick to what is familiar, our thought patterns sometimes keeps us isolated and not willing to go where we have not been before. When the body and the mind is disconnected it is difficult to trust and start again in life.

Where do we go from here? Although I hear of many people complaining about how things are more complicated and difficult today, I believe otherwise. We are very much dancing in the chaos of life; this is where changes occur. After all the confusion comes calm and order. It is like a defragmentation process of eliminating what is clogging the system and starting afresh with a system that works efficiently.

Since the world got reconstructed after World War II the planet has gone though many transformations. Some part of it is constantly being destroyed whereas other parts are being recreated. We are constantly rebuilding ourselves and our planet by tapping into the abundance that is already there. Although nations from some parts of the world are still trying to destroy each other the majority of human beings only want peace and harmony. Most are learning to negotiate so to live in a more unified way. People tend to travel frequently these days and learn from different cultures, embracing new ways of appreciating the world we live in. Although there have many major issues that still affect the world, on a global scheme people from different countries tend to collectively work towards a more peaceful world. We are not so separated as nations but instead we want to connect in a way that collective we can create that peaceful world that we so desire.

Objections and responses:

We have to keep traditions.

Yes, some traditions are worth keeping but some have to go if we want to progress in creating a more unified world.

We have to protect our country from those who want to invade it.

People are constantly moving around in the world today. We now realise that the world belongs to everyone and this is how we are gradually breaking down the barriers.

The terrorists are causing a lot of havoc in the world. We have to stop them.

We can only stop the terrorists if we are united and work towards for what we stand for – unity in the world.

3 actions to take as a result of reading this chapter:
1. Looking at your purpose in the world and how to contribute to it.
2. Connecting with others and collaborating to make the world a better place.
3. Be instrumental in shifting things in your world one day at a time to impact the whole world.

A conversation with Rudran Brannock

A healer who healed himself from emphysema.

Christiane: I was talking to this young guy yesterday, only about 16 or so, and he's saying, 'I don't believe God actually allows all this suffering to take place and if he does then he's not a good God. How would he allow these things to happen?'

Rudran: Morality is a line of development and that line of development, when it stops being separate. Morality seems to morph into compassion, and I don't mean just an empathic kind of thing that people call compassion or altruism. I'm talking about that rich, deep compassion where I see you are part of what I am and your suffering is my suffering, and your joys are my joys and so I can no longer say, stand in judgement as a separate person and go, you are right and wrong and good and bad and so on, it's not possible, because it's too intimate, it's too resonate. That's how it seems to me that my morality has grown up and had gone past good and bad and come to a place of resonance and compassion and that's how that part of it seems to me.

Thinking can give you doors to walk through, but you have to walk through them psychologically, you have to pass through the doors that thought can help create for you, but thought can only create. You know the biggest intellectual can only create a hall full of doorways. And you have to walk through those doors. That's just how that is.

Christiane: I think as we experience life and as we experience the lessons that we have to learn then we discover that we gain something each time.
Rudran: I think we get more expanded as we go, too. We get bigger.

Christiane: I wouldn't say knowledge, but it's like the intelligence. Have another piece of that intelligence that's available to us, and yet at the very beginning we don't know that it exists and then we find, oh, there is something more than I thought was there and that's also this intelligence is very much a part of who we are, it's within us but we don't know it's there. Does that make sense?
Rudran: I agree with you. I see it as intelligence also, I think. Any part that I refer to as me is my spirit, that's how I think of it. And I don't mean that collections of connections and experiences that makes this big kind of whirlwind of connections. I'm talking about when I'm in the Chi of it and I can feel the whole movement of the energy of life in others and I can feel myself directing my Chi and receiving, I can feel that and I call that part my spirit. And the egoic part of me I call that my cultural self, my ego.

Beliefs and opinions and thoughts and emotions and desires and all of that, we filter it through this whole matrix of the past, of yesterday really. And of course there are times without filters as well. Like there are times when that whole egoic sense is just not there. Like suddenly if I see a drop dead gorgeous sunset and I just open and all that stuff is not there and all there is beauty, there's no filter in that. If I'm making love with my woman and something happens and some moment and all the divisions vanish and there's no filters in there.

Christiane: Yeah, because that's the present moment, and when we live in the present moment there's only bliss.

Rudran: I'm not sure whether that's true. I can be really present with a broken leg and there's nothing very blissful about that.

Christiane: But then you can accept, instead of making this situation wrong, you can say, okay I've got a broken leg.

Rudran: That's right. I think its acceptance also and not identifying it. Not identifying with the pain, not identifying with the body. And I do... it seems to me from what I know of enlightened people that they reach a point where everything is blissful for them and I don't think it's simply a matter of being present, it's how deeply you are in the present, I suspect. Because I understand that I can be very present with walking but if I'm much more subtle in that moment, I actually am present with a lot more, because I can actually perceive a lot more and so I think, and these enlightened people to me, I think they're just fully mature human beings, that's how I view it and I think from what they say, that they live a life of bliss.

And I think one thing I heard from one of Buddha's answers, when somebody said, what is enlightenment? And he would give lots of answers to that question, he got asked that a lot. One of his answers was, constant insight. And I understand that ... and I know what insight is like. When I have a whole body insight it's this full energy event that goes on and to be constantly like that, would take extraordinary energy and I also know what it's like, because I've been studying tantric sexuality for some time.

Christiane: I haven't really explored that area yet.

Rudran: What they call tantric sexuality or sacred sexuality or kadoshka seem to me they're simply an adult version of sexuality, and when you become conscious of the energy of your sexuality and you move with it consciously, then you enter into this realm they call Tantra or sacred sexuality. And we give it special names I think because our entire culture is very adolescent or preadolescent and so most of what happens, everything from politics to university teaching and I think it's all very young.

I've been studying my Chi, for a very long time, for nearly 40 years and the way that the energy moves, to be conscious of that, is to be an adult. And people are not conscious of it, they're still struggling to get through adolescence, they're still living in this world of think emote, think emote, think emote, it's like this ego cycle thing that goes on and they're not dropping underneath all that to this deep, deep feeling where the spirit is much more easily seen, the action. That to me is adulthood.

Christiane: What interests me is that what you're talking about is like we're just very young, and did you say with that we haven't come into adulthood yet? Or what was it that you said?

Rudran: Well generally speaking if we talk about adulthood we talk about the end of adolescence, normally. We talk about childhood, adolescence, adulthood. When we come into adolescence, it's when our sexual energy starts to become external, so we can create babies, our bodies firm up, the bones get hard and we develop the physical and the mental and emotional capacity to be independent adults within the culture. That is that period of adolescence, so it's not simply a physical body coming somewhere, or the sexual energy coming, it is also the emotional line of development as well, goes through a period of adolescence and the intellectual line of development, like learning to abstract reasoning and all of those things that are part of it and so our sexual line of development as well.

The way that I see that is we begin our sexual adolescence and from that moment we can create babies. Once a woman starts bleeding or a man can produce sperm, have erections, in that place we can have babies, we can produce more human beings. And then any adolescent can do that. You don't have to be an adult for that.

Christiane: Once your organs are active you can produce babies.

Rudran: Yes, you can produce babies. That's the adolescent period. And so when a person becomes an adult, they become independent. What is adulthood to me is a movement into independence. I become physically independent, I can work for a living. I'm sexually independent, that means I'm no longer dependant on other people for my sexuality.

Just have a look at the level of morality around sexuality, it's a very repressed, 50 or 60 years ago, but it's still a very repressed sexual society. That's what I mean adulthood in that line of development, emotionally a person becomes independent, when they no longer have emotions that require other people. So for example guilt is a culturally evoked emotion, whereas when I can discriminate the difference between remorse, remorse is when I have done something, I know I've wronged you and in that knowledge, straight away I want to make amends.

Guilt on the other hand is something cultural and is based around right and wrong and good and bad and based around social morality. When guilt comes to an end, jealousy comes to an end. Envy. These all require other people. And so when those things come to an end I'm in my emotional adulthood.

And so each line of development is the independence that comes, like intellectually. To be intellectually independent means that I can think for myself. It means that I can use clear thinking and not be affected by emotional events. External to me, so there's a lot of people got very cranky because Donald Trump won the election and there's all this emotional childish stuff going on and it's really easy to me, I can feel the energy, it's very clear to me why many working class people supported him, it was very clear and yet all these people and yet all the intellectuals are making theories, on talk shows, writing books and they're doing all this stuff all based on this emotional thing and they can't think very clearly because they're so emotionally conditioned in all these beliefs and all of that. They're not intellectually independent, their intellect is still at an adolescent level, that's how I see that.

Also spiritually as you say we get brought up with a religion, we get brought up with beliefs and all of that and then when we reach adolescence, like the 16 year old you mentioned, he's saying, well I don't believe that a God could allow this suffering and so this questioning comes about and then eventually a person starts to become not so judgemental of others, starts to become more compassionate and all of that. That person starts to resonate with the energy of the other, they resonate with the tree, with the stone, with the traffic, with the people in the house and so on.

This resonance with is very different from, I'm separate in here and you're separate in there and I get information from you and I judge you accordingly to the information I'm getting and all of that idea of life, made of around separation starts coming to an end.

That's how I see adulthood.

Christiane: You were talking about enlightenment and the people you know, the people who are enlightened.
Rudran: Well I've only ever met one. That's Ama, do you know her? They call her the Hugging Saint. She goes around the world hugging people. She's a very traditional Hindu way but she herself is not Hindu or anything. She does those forms, because that's the culture she grew in and so she goes and does all the festivals and holidays that the Hindus do because that's her country and so on, but she's one of these people like Buddha, then Jesus. I've read of quite a few; Yogananda, Muktinanda, a lot of Indian people.

In Australia, Barry Long was one guy here, inspiring people ... in all societies, there's many. And I can't really say what they're like, because I only met one.

Christiane: You met her?
Rudran: I met her yes. I go and see her every time she comes to Australia, for the last 20 years, I go and see her, I do retreats with her and all that.

Christiane: If everybody is the mirror image of who you are ... Whatever you like in them is whatever you've got within yourself and whatever you don't like about them it's something you've got to look at and see whether there's anything to transform.

Rudran: I discovered that whenever I didn't like a quality in someone, it was because I had that quality in me hidden. I also found that if there was some quality in someone that I really admired and I actually had that quality that was nascent in myself.

I used to go and hang out with those people, if they had qualities I admired. And so I grew up very quickly from that. It's a great way to grow up, to hang out with people you admire.

Christiane: Can you tell me a little bit about the workshops that you do?

Rudran: I do quite a few. I've done a lot of work with men over the years. I do men's workshops and the main workshop I do there now is called Advanced Men's Business.

And I run a workshop called Awakening the Ecstatic Body and this is about awakening the animal part of us, because we are born with certain animal propensities and desires and so on and it's the job of the culture to take that animal part of us and bend it in a direction that the society wants, so you learn how to survive within society and all of that. And when we are living a more close to nature life when our culture is close to nature, then the animal part of us flows naturally, the culture has not got all these constrictions against it.

Christiane: When you talk about the hara, does this have anything to do with the tantric energy?

Rudran: Normally they don't teach it that way, because tantric sexuality as it's taught is only really about the sexual energy. As it pertains to being in a relationship and desire, that's all. If you want to use that energy for something else, you need to do something else. And that something else is to move it from the hara, so that is why I teach that. But in my sexual life I keep hara a lot during sexuality anyway and a lot of different things happen, so I've had a lot of experiences that normal tantric people and tantric teachers, they don't have those experiences, because they don't keep hara.

I also show how to raise the animal body, because our animal selves get conditioned by culture and the further we get away from a culture that's connected with nature, the more that animal energy we have gets repressed. And so we lose that energy. I've needed to find that more in me for my own healing, I've had to release that energy so I can use it. And there's a lot of ways, a lot of shamanic ways to do that, but the simplest way is through yawning and stretching the way that animals do. This is the way they keep resetting their bodies. You know when we have a really satisfying yawn in the morning?

It's called pandiculation. When we do yoga, we stretch this [gesturing on video]. As I stretch this, that's yoga. When I do this, that's pandiculation. And if you pandiculate your whole body and you do it as part of your morning routine, then all this animal energy that you've had repressed for most of your life comes available to you, and you can use that energy for whatever you want, you can use it for healing.

The other element is to discover the masculine and feminine dance of the breath. The feminine breath is internal, masculine breath is external. If you have a breath that focuses on the in breath, just let the out breath fall away, that's a feminine breath, a surrender breath. That's what they use in rebirthing and these types of modalities. Breaths that focus on the out breath, like in yoga, we do this breath called bellows breath. Which is a really masculine breath, fire breath. You breathe through the nose and all you do is push the air out quickly and let the air come in on its own. So all you're focussing on the out breath and you go ... (breathing) Like that. That's what we call a bellows breath or a fire breath and that's a masculine breath. So when you learn how to dance with that, that also brings energy and helps you focus energy. There's a very masculine breath where you make a small sound in the back of your throat and you breathe in with this sound, so you go (breathing). Can you hear that? Like Darth Vader in Star Wars. That's a very controlling breath and you get to control your energy. When you build your energy and draw your energy, draw your sexual energy, you pandiculate and you might want to control that, you send that energy somewhere and you use the controlling breath for that. When you just want to open to what's there, say you might have past issues or something, you want to open you use your surrender breath. Which is like the rebirth you go ... (breathing). Like this. Just like a sigh, a surrender.

This workshop came about because of my self-healing. Because I'd had the type A influenza virus about 10 years ago, after that I had post-viral fatigue. And it went on for a very long time and the doctors were saying, 'You've got the classic symptoms of depression, do you want some anti-depressant drugs?

This way of looking at it isn't what I need to do and so I went to this Chinese herbalist and got herbs and eventually went to an Ayurvedic practitioner. I had already been doing yoga and breathing, but it got so bad at one point that I had to make absolute discipline to do five minutes of yoga in the morning and five minutes of yoga in the afternoon. Just five minutes and sometimes I dozed off on the yoga mat.

At night I was sweating enough to make my t-shirt wet. Then in the day I would have one hour sleeps between 3-6 times during the day. That's how fatigued I was. But eventually it got a bit better, but it wasn't until eventually I said to myself, look I've been studying all this yoga, all this aikido, Tantra, I did all these things, I must be able to heal myself. So I started to experiment a lot with my energy and I eventually got this one where I just told you about where I draw my sexual energy into my hara, draw my energy down the top of my spine in my hara, this is a breath that they call uniting the heaven and earth in the lower abdomen.

But I was drawing my sexual energy into there as well. Sexual energy is a big energy; I want you to use it for healing. Not the Ayurveda and the Chinese guy said that I had difficulty with my adrenals and also with my spleen. So what I did was I drew all this energy into my hara and I wrapped it around my body and the first time I did that it felt like my lower body was encased in a womb.

It just felt wonderful and so I started to do that every day and after two weeks I was noticeably better. A year ago or so I went to a workshop on TRE, trauma release exercises, and that's all about tremoring, allowing your body to tremor. Now I've been practising how to tremor my body, how can I tremor this finger, that finger, so I've been very interested in all of that.

But what happened a couple of years ago, I'd started to get arthritis and so I changed my diet, alkalised my diet as you do. That helped a great deal.

Christiane: So how do you alkalise your diet?
Rudran: Well you stop eating bacon and eggs, start eating leafy greens and drink fresh lemon in water, first thing in the morning, I've been doing that for a very long time. That's one way. Also if you drink coconut water in the morning. Different foods take a different level of acid relationship in the body. Red meat, for example, you've got to put a lot of acid in your body to digest it. So it acidifies your body. What acidifies your body is really about how much acid you put into your stomach from the food. So fruit, for example, doesn't take as much and fish doesn't take as much as red meat, but it's still very acidic for me. So I talk about acidic for me, that's what they talk about, not the acid in the food itself, although some food has lactic acid in it like meat, so that comes in your body, too.

To alkalise your body you would start off in the morning with lemon water and maybe eat fruit and then just slowly build in and you'd stop eating red meat altogether, stop having coffee, tea, all these things that acidify the body and you stop having that stuff if you need to alkalise your body.

Two and a half years ago I got diagnosed with emphysema. And so straight away I went into doing these lung exercises and downloaded things from the Internet, yogic breathing techniques, did all that a lot of experimenting. I was getting up early in the morning and spending two, two and a half hours every morning on my own healing and I did various things, too, like there's things you can do with healing light, bring in healing light and so on.

I did that just about every day for about seven months and then I got the specialist to do all the tests again, and he said, oh you haven't got it.

Christiane: So what brought that on? Emphysema?
Rudran: I used to smoke cigarettes, but I was also raised in a mining town in Mount Isa and when there was no wind, the smoke would pour down the stack and all over the town like they're smelting lead and copper and all that stuff.

Christiane: So that's remained in your body for all that time?
Rudran: I think probably, well it might, I'm not too sure, but it certainly wouldn't have made the lungs any healthier. And I had also had very bad asthma and bronchitis when I was a boy as well. I actually died in an ambulance from complications of asthma and bronchitis and they gave me a shot of adrenaline in the heart to bring me back.

Christiane: Wow! You've come from a long way.
Rudran: My memory of that is very different. What I remember is the image of my memory and it's different to having an experience in these places that they call spiritual realms, the mind puts into an imagery that is understandable. My memory of it was I was in this cave, there was a big hole, a big long tunnel in a cave and I was in the lip of this big hole, leaning on my elbows in the floor of the cave and there's this big hole going way down into the earth and I'm leaning there and there's these beings of golden light standing on these big rocks. And they were saying, do you want to go back and finish your purpose? Finish your job? It doesn't matter, you don't have to, it will get done anyway, but it's just easiest if you do it.

And then I sort of reluctantly agreed and I let go, I remember flying down this and I woke up and I can't remember where I was but there was all this psychic stuff and it was just too much and I closed down and then I woke up in an oxygen tent.

That's my memory as a three year old.

Christiane: You were three then?

Rudran: I was three years old, yeah.

Christiane: Whatever is in this world, it's all an illusion. And it's not what we think it is. It's the only way our mind comprehends it and so just hearing your version of what it was, so that was just really all to do with you, your mission and what you're here for and what you're meant to do and whereas if we go back connecting with people every day on a human level, everything is totally different, it's like a different story, isn't it?

And when we delve into who we really are and our self, and only you call that your soul or your spirit.

Rudran: Yeah, I can use the word soul, but I don't usually. Words get loaded with meaning and also I can't really discriminate yet. They talk about everything being made of spirit, people talk like that. And they say we're like a droplet of spirit, and then you get a drop out of an ocean of water, the drop is itself, but it's still a part of the whole. They talk about it like that. And I can't discriminate between when I'm in that, I don't have any discrimination between what is me or spirit and what is other of spirit and I can't. Apparently you're supposed to be able to but I don't know how to do that.

If it's true, I'll find out some time.

Christiane: So what do you think of when you hear that we're made of atoms? The human body is made of atoms.

Rudran: Well, that's also true. See the energies of which atoms are made, atoms are made of subatomic particles and those subatomic particles are made of energy. That's what modern physics tells us. Everything is essentially made of energy. And I think that you get all this energy it's a certain shape, like the energy gets a pattern. This is what we call matter. That's how I tend to see it.

And I'm a cultural being, and so most of my cultural self is to do with thought and one of the big traps is identifying the content of my own thought. My thought is not the thing that it represents, it's just not. It's only in here. It's only in here. And when I believe in it, like Byron Katie says, don't believe in your thoughts, it's a waste of time. If I believe in my thoughts, it is really stupid, it's very young, and it's a very undeveloped mind that believes that its thoughts are reality.

Christiane: Your thought is really a collective of whatever you see and hear and you put it in a story, don't you?
Rudran: That's exactly so. And it's made out of the past. Made out of beliefs and opinions and experiences. That's what the story is made of and that's the filter I look at the world and it's a complete illusion.

Christiane: Because everything we see, hear and believe from the past, everything that happens, like every thought that happens, happened a minute ago is already passed anyway.
Rudran: It's already past, that's right.

Christiane: Which means it's all made from the past.
Rudran: All made of the past. Totally.

Christiane: And sometimes we try to identify what is our mind and what is our thought and where is our mind located and where our thoughts are located and whether to believe your thought, but also because our brain is actually governing a lot of our thoughts, as part of our mind does, but it's also to, once we give it instructions, to do a goal or to do something that we want to achieve, then it's there to serve us.

Whereas unguided it will just use what's been stored from the past and will just make a story out of that.
Rudran: That's right. That's my experience as well.

Christiane: And then it will cling to whatever the mind is manufacturing as a story and then most of it will go live it. And I suppose this is what you mean by like a not grown up mind, it's just a childish mind that allows, which we actually surround our will or wanting to do something for ourselves to what our mind tells us is right. And what it has seen and what it has believed from what's been information that's been given to it.
Rudran: It's a very poor master. It needs to be the servant, not the master.

Christiane: This is where a lot of people tend to get stuck in. And the idea is not to get trapped into it, because even when we are and if we're sick and diagnosed with any illness or anything that we actually get affected by and if we allow our thoughts to govern what should happen, then we're doomed, aren't we?

Rudran: Yeah and all of the enlightened people talk about all of this constantly. Buddha would be saying, you are what you think. He's not saying to change your thoughts to something else and believe something else, which is what mostly they talk about in our society, what he's saying is what happens in the absence of thought? Who are you without thought?

All of the teachers, Judaeo Christian, who I've been reading for a very long time, and Osho and Ama, they're always talking about this thing, thought. I even think there's a mistranslation in the Bible, I think when Jesus is saying, 'Why take ye thought for raiment? Consider the lilies of the valley, how they grow'. And generally Christians look at this to say, 'What good are clothes?' Look at the lilies of the valley, that's how they look at it. I look at it as Jesus saying, 'Why do you take thought for clothing'. You know? Why take thought for raiment? That's what I think he's referring to. Why do you clothe yourself in thought?

Rudran Brannock

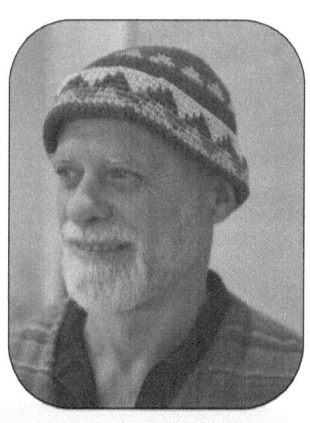

Founder and visionary of The Joining, a gathering for the coming together of the Masculine and the Feminine both internally and externally in our relationships and occasional consulting editor for Living Now magazine on matters masculine and feminine, Rudran Brannock is in the business of conscious culture.

> 'Because the world is in peril and you and I are going to save her. Not just the world without, but the world within.'
> – Rudran Brannock

Employing advanced techniques and processes – some rather ancient and some on the cutting edge, Rudran works on three levels: supporting development with individuals; facilitation of workshops; and through the creation of sustainable cultural forms.

Currently heading the Culture and Gender Department of the Sustainability Research Institute, Rudran is working on multiple projects, including the publication of his first book.

Afterword

I appreciate sharing this book with you. It has taken me a long while to get here.

I have had so many questions answered for myself while writing this book. For many years I have been asking myself questions about life, people, events, and what the future holds. Human beings have challenges because it is all part of our growth and how we can evolve on this planet. The planet has been through so many transformations already. Delving into the history of planet Earth we find how battles and wars of the past centuries have been instrumental in causing a lot of destruction and suffering to this planet and its inhabitants.

Now our task is to save the planet so we can save humanity. We have to start with ourselves, our health, and wellbeing. There is a great task ahead of us because it is not about us only. We have to start thinking in a way of community again to help others heal themselves.

I keep going back to the Oriental philosophy. Had I not been exposed to it, I would have been living on medication permanently by now. Oriental principles have the most precise way of restoring health and wellbeing because they had their wisdom passed to them by many sages from the East so many centuries BC; that includes Confucius and Lao-tse.

I am offering you, the reader, a lot of clues in this book to start your own research so you can answer your own questions and become your own healer. As I have undertaken the path to healing humanity and the planet, I invite you to join me in healing yourself to help restore our Earth. I feel that this book is only a draft of what I wanted to cover. I still have so many questions in my head but I am running out of time to get this book to you.

Life is a big mystery! Unless we keep asking many questions, we cannot get the answers. When we share our experiences it seems to unlock something in others around us. If we isolate ourselves we completely cut ourselves off from others. Many use religion as an authority to act a certain way or to justify their rights. Religion is meant to create unity. It is only when we stand united we can create joy and happiness for ourselves and others.

References and Other Reading

M Emoto, *The True Power of Water* (Atria Books 2003, 2005)

K.H. Albertine et al, *Pocket Anatomicas Body Atlas* (Global Book Publishing 2007, 2008, 2009)

D. Chopra M.D., *Perfect Health: The Complete Mind/Body Guide* (Bantam Books 1990)

D. Chopra, *Power, Freedom, and Grace: Living from the Source of Lasting Happiness* (Amber-Allen Publishing, Inc. 2006)

T Dedopulos, *Kabbalah, An Introduction to the Esoteric Heart of Jewish Mysticism* (Penguin Books, Australia 2005)

M Hattstein, *The Story of World Religions* (Könemann)

P.J. D'Adamo, *Eat Right 4 Your Type* (Century, London 2001)

G. Ohsawa, *Zen Macrobiotics* (The Ohsawa Foundation 1965)

About the Author

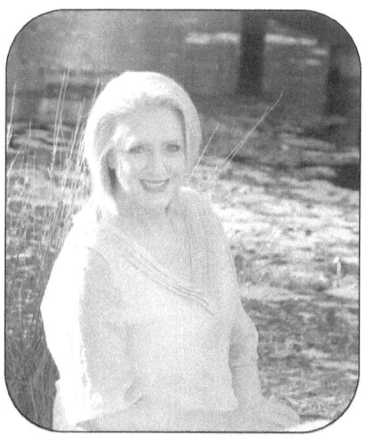

Christiane moved to Australia from Mauritius in 1971. Two months after arriving in Australia, she started a career with the Department of Defence. During her 25 years with Defence she worked in finance, logistics, and Information Technology. During the time that she was managing the Military Library in Moorebank Christiane studied an Associate Diploma in Arts, specialising in Library. In 1996, she started a small business in Soft Furnishing and Decor. She enjoyed embellishing some notable homes in the most affluent parts of Sydney.

Christiane was in a very destructive marriage for many years, being a victim of domestic violence. She felt humiliated and did not want to share what she was going through. It took a long time to get her life together again. She met a coach who helped her get her power back. She then had the courage to end her marriage.

When Christiane came to the Gold Coast in 2004, she felt that she wanted to contribute more to humanity. In 2007, Christiane embarked on an intense coaching training programme which lasted for 12 months. During that time she worked closely with a Master Coach. This was the foundation for her total transformation and in realising her dreams to be of service to humanity.

Christiane is very connected to health and wellbeing. In April 2014, she succumbed to a slipped disc and the doctor's diagnosis was heavy painkillers and impending surgery. With sheer determination she started investigating alternative solutions that got her some amazing results. With intense physiotherapy, acupuncture, and osteopath treatments she finally got the normal use of her limbs again. She no longer required surgery nor medication.

In October 2015, Christiane's health was challenged again as she was diagnosed with Type II diabetes. Determined to restore her health she rigidly followed a blood type diet that she had been following casually for five years. She implemented a tough routine of daily walks and meditation. She was able to get off her medications within a few months.

Her passion is to educate committed people willing to restore their health naturally. She follows the Zen Macrobiotic principles that have helped her maintain a balanced and healthy life. Christiane believes that people can avoid surgery and avoid living permanently on medical prescription if they choose to.

Her ultimate goal is to promote vitality, longevity, and natural healing.

Contact Christiane

Email:christianeongc@gmail.com

Health Dynamics Packages

Product and Services	Silver	Gold	Platinum
Free On-Line Course	✓	✓	✓
6 Months Coaching	✓	✓	✓
Half Day Workshop	✓	✓	✓
5 Goal Cards	✓	✓	✓
Meditation Cushion	✓	✓	✓
Free Meditation with the Flute CD	✓	✓	✓
Free eBook	✓	✓	✓
Access to Facebook Group	✓	✓	✓
1 Free Massage Session		✓	✓
2 Hour Healing Session		✓	✓
5 Steps to Transforming Your Life		✓	✓
Health Dynamics 2 Day Retreat			✓
Invitation to 'End of Year Reunion'			✓
12 Month Mentoring & Coaching			✓
12 Month Health Monitor Programme			✓
1 Pamper Session with Essential Oils			✓

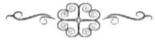

Blockage Release Session - 90 Minutes Consultation

- Are you having problems putting your goals together?
- Are you having a headful of ideas and can't get started?
- Are you wanting feedback on a few things you have been stuck on and need a helping hand?
- Are you feeling overwhelmed and can't face it all by yourself at the moment?
- Are you dealing with some upset that you are having difficulty letting go?
- Are you dealing with relationship issues that have you going back to the past?
- Are you feeling resentment, regrets or any negative emotions playing on your mind

This session includes:

- 30 minutes meditation
- 15 to 30 minutes healing
- 30 to 45 minutes of consultation

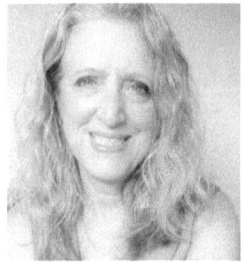

Christiane seems to have been a coach all her life. She is interested in what people are dealing with and endevours herself to have them look at what is not working to start removing what is in the way to create a new space for anything new and exciting in their life.

Whatever you are at, Christiane will help assist you in rediscovering yourself and find your special magic again. When meeting your next challenge you will be well-equippped to handle the toughest situation.

Now is the time to have a chat. Take advantage of your 15 minutes FREE consultation.

Email: christianeongc@gmail.com

www.ingramcontent.com/pod-product-compliance
Lightning Source LLC
Chambersburg PA
CBHW030329080526
44584CB00012B/786